For Kris,

Because sexuality is intimate, unique and personal and deserves so much more than just a fleeting glance.

Sensuality without love is a sin;

love without sensuality is worse than a sin.

- Jose Bergamin

Introduction

I'll make this easy for you. Your main aphrodisiac oils are:

- Rose
- Jasmine
- Sandalwood
- Ylang Ylang

If you are looking for an essential oils recipe book, then there's your cookie cutter mix. No need to buy the book, take that information for free. These are oils guaranteed to get you in the mood.

But aromatherapy is capable of so much more. The reason my libido falls will be different from yours. There are myriad reasons why people become frigid or feel unable to submit to sex. For many, desire may be there, but the mind is not so keen. Ejaculation comes too early, orgasms fail to erupt, and sex can get very painful.

I've given you aphrodisiac oils for free, but what if getting in the mood isn't your issue. What if something else keeps getting in the way. Well, then essential oils can most certainly help, but only inside of the concept of aromatherapy and that's a very different thing from just a couple of drops of aphrodisiac essential oil.

Aromatherapy addresses each person (or in the case of this book, the couple) as individuals. It's about peeling back the layers, to find where the problem lies. Even issues like pain during intercourse, or impotence, that are most definitely physical manifestations, may have root causes in stress, trauma, or rage. Viagra will get the erection, but aromatherapy can help remove the source.

Sexual relations are often fraught with cultural overlays and history brought to the bed. Institutions like marriage place huge psychological pressure on couples, profoundly interwoven with perceived expectations to perform, not only between the sheets but also financially, and with childrearing and cooking. If a partner feels they might not keeping up their half of the bargain, then often their feelings will become confused into sexual dysfunction too.

Sometimes conditioned attitudes and feelings about sex have enormous disparities in a relationship. Men are conditioned that virility and being a successful man depends on how many conquests he can make. A woman, however, is told if she has too much sex, she is loose. These inequalities have power to create silent rifts in partnerships. How many times a week then is appropriate for them? Immediately, living within those parameters, one lover often feels frustrated and the other ashamed. Yet talking about it can be impossible for some.

As we age, naturally, erections soften, and vaginas start to dry. Culturally, we are asked to take a pill or see a counsellor if our libido starts to wane. The 1970's sexual revolution did much to liberate women, but as a bi-product it created a new conditioning about sex. Somehow, in the glitz and glamour of equality and choice, sex has been isolated from love, almost as if emotions are outdated and inconvenient.

Yet, as humans, feelings and emotional connection are what connect us with source. What if, sex was more than just about the physical body? What if "successful sex" whatever that might look like, depended on emotions and spiritual communion bringing us closer together in a more intimate state of union.

Well, then often confidence needs to build, and security requires a little work. Forgiveness needs to happen for a new sense of openness and vulnerability to take anger's place.

So easy to write on paper, but with neurochemistry jamming heartache into your memories over and over again, incredibly difficult to do. Recollections of hurt and rage scream in your face every time bed linen touches bare skin and, while you might not feel that fury, your body's reaction shuts your lover out again.

A vicious and hateful cycle...

What if I told you those neurochemicals can be changed? That essential oils encourage the release of emotional and physical pain. That by some strange quirk of nature, a plant might just be your salvation from this hell and find a way to bring you and your soul mate back together again. What would you say to that...?

Sounds good right?

Step inside my fragrant boudoir and, for the sexually distressed and the merely lusty, there are many erotic secrets concealed within.

Take my hand...gently, of course. That's how I like it.

Contents

Chapter 1 The Physiology of Sex

Let's start with some science. Normally, I'd begin with anatomy, but I think within the remit of this book, we can say we know the important bits that do what, (or in some cases don't do it) so we'll skip that.

Sexual Dysfunction

Dysfunction falls into four categories.

- Desire - loss of either interest in sex of a fall in sexual interest
- Arousal - Unable to become physically aroused or excited during sexual relations
- Orgasm - absence of orgasm or a delay of it
- Pain disorders - pain during intercourse

Sexual Drive

Science shows us that men's and women's sexual drives are differently wired. Men are more likely to be spontaneously aroused and respond to visual cues, consequently they respond well to sexy outfits, pornography and they masturbate more. Many men report being so turned on by the scent of a woman, that the aroma alone might be enough to make them come, leading scientists to speculate whether they may have olfactory receptors a-tuned to the scent of oestrogen, making them alert as soon as they smell a new strain.

A woman is less likely to become aroused spontaneously, her desire being more adapted to her circumstances. So, for many women the adage of wanting to be wined and dined is exactly accurate.

Men have no need to feel emotionally connected to their partner, whereas a woman is more likely to feel desire from some emotional connection to a person.

Women are twice as likely to go off sex and will usually attribute this to poor mental and physical health in general, feeling emotionally distant to their partner, and not being able to communicate with their partner about sex.

Men are perhaps a trickier breed, to analyse, given that many perceive a connection between their sexual drive and their power as a man, and thus might be less likely to admit it has waned. Studies of those who have commented, however, showed "that lack of interest was *more* commonly reported by men who had recently masturbated, but *less* commonly reported by women who had done so."

Interestingly, men seem not to be very perturbed by having young children in the house, something that radically affects a woman's drive. (Is it sexist to say that's a telling statement?)

Where a decline in sexual drive is most definitely related to age, and it drops earlier in women than men, it does not affect the ability to orgasm, which continues until way after you are 90 years old!

Sexual drive can be affected by any number of things, from stress to hormonal imbalance and medications.

An interesting phenomenon has been identified in rats (and here I am talking about rodents not cheating men!) that shows that their libido will drop with long term partners, but then if a new female enters the mix, the furry fiend will suddenly perk up and look interested, even if he is still surrounded by females he has previously had sex with. More, the male, who would normally need a refractory period (i.e a bit of a rest after orgasm) can suddenly perform immediately.

It seems this is common behaviour amongst male mammals and to a lesser degree, females. Amusingly, this is referred to as the Coolidge Effect, after a remark The First Lady, Grace Coolidge, wife to the 30th President of the United States, made while being shown around a government farm. She noticed one rooster having an impressive number of conquests. She enquired how often that happened and was told by the attendant, "Dozens of times each day." Mrs. Coolidge smiled and whispered, "Tell that to the President when he comes by." Upon being told, the President Coolidge wanted to know, "Same hen every time?" The reply came, "Oh, no, Mr. President, a different hen every time." President Coolidge quipped: "Tell *that* to Mrs. Coolidge."

To balance the tale, it is noticed that women will also often gravitate to flirt with new males in the group.

So, we know that sexual interest doesn't necessarily match to being paired with a partner. Biology literally forces us to peek outside of the relationship to sniff for something different. Perhaps predictably keeping the light off for every interlude, is playing into nature's hands. To play biochemistry at its own game, maybe we need to change things up a bit every now and then.

Sometimes though sex drive is affected by our life style and we do have some influence over these.

Medications

Blood pressure tablets and ACE Inhibitors both play havoc with sexual function. It may be worth asking your doctor to try you on a different brand. Likewise, chronic conditions such as arthritis and diabetes negatively impact sexuality. Depression affects how we feel generally and lowers libido and interest in sex, however anti-depressants can do the same. SSRI medications especially disturb sexual function. I talk about the relationship between rose, SSRI and treating loss of male sexual function extensively in my book Rose Goddess Medicine. You might want to cross reference there.

Sleep

Paradoxically, the one thing sex steals from us – sleep – will ultimately reek its revenge. Sleep deprivation eventually affects sex drive. Sleep apnea, in particular, is proven to drive testosterone down. Men with low levels of testosterone often exhibit low libido, and so drive and sexual activity both take the strain.

A blend of thyme, lemon, peppermint, and eucalyptus has been proven to reduce snoring. Add valerian and spikenard for a peaceful night's sleep.

Restless Legs Syndrome

Research shows that men who endure restless legs syndrome are at higher risk of erectile dysfunction. A man who experiences five disturbed nights a month is more than 50% more likely to develop problems with dysfunction and that rises even more for men who have a greater number of restless nights.

RLS might be one of aromatherapy's greatest success stories. Easily treated with a mix of Epsom Salts and Clary Sage essential oil in the bath.

Zdravetz *(Geranium macrorrhizum)* essential oil is aphrodisiac, antispasmodic and encourages sleep. Catnip *(Nepeta cataria)* too, is a wonderfully peaceful lullaby.

Age

Naturally, our bodies change, and it is normal for men's libido to drop at around 60-65. It takes more mature men longer to become aroused, to climax and ejaculate. Their penis will take longer to harden and will not be as hard as it was when he was younger. Jasmine oil is very useful for all of these issues.

Stress

Stress directly affects hormonal levels and the neurochemistry that drives our sexuality forwards, but it also narrows the arteries too, affecting blood flow to a man's erection. Vaso-relaxant oils, reversing this action, such as geranium, rose and bergamot are perhaps some of the most popular and easiest to use in aphrodisiac blends.

In this book, we take it as read that stress exists in every relationship, but science tells us that stress will impact on sexual drive even if there are no psychological issues or relationship problems. In other words, just because your partner has gone off sex, certainly doesn't mean it has anything to do with you. It doesn't mean they no longer love or need you, life might just feel too hard right now.

Poor body image

Scientists have proven a direct relationship between a woman's feelings about how she looks, and how satisfying her experience of sex will be. At each stage of the sexual cycle, from desire to climax, negative thought patterns impede sexual experience.

Analysis of studies data reveals sexual satisfaction can be predicted by how high a person's body esteem is, since they have fewer distracting thoughts about their appearance during sex, so are more focused on enjoyment..

Yuzu, sandalwood and vetiver oils are amazing for centring the thoughts and helping you to be more present in the moment.

Negative Sexual History
Clearly a history of abuse or negative sexual experiences will also affect how likely you are to want to be intimate.

Arousal Disorders

Sexual Arousal Disorder
Here we have a lack of sexual response to sexual stimulation, whether that be mental or emotional, or to physical stimuli. So, for some women, kissing, dancing close or reading an erotic tale will not cause that tell-tale tingling feeling and throbbing as blood flows to their sex.

Conversely, some women are entirely aroused by the more emotional and mental stimulus but feel nothing when their genitals are touched, or worse only feel pain.

The same sorts of issues tend to be causal, as with libido issues. Oestrogen levels, feelings of intimacy, distracting thoughts or evaluating one's overall sexual performance can all get in the way. Physiological issues such as skin changes in the vulva, thinning and drying of the vagina or even an age related decline in a woman's testosterone levels can bring about these changes.

Therapies tend to rely on creating a more romantic setting for sexual relations, as well as learning how to communicate what feels good and what doesn't. Often wooing much more slowly and experimenting without touching the genitals helps to relax and focus the attention on what turns you on. This change in dynamics aids feelings of intimacy and trust which can often be transformative in these conditions,

Oils such as clary sage, jasmine, Zdravetz (*Geranium macrorrhizum*) and roman camomile are excellent antispasmodics and can be used well as creams inserted into the vagina. Clary sage also mimics the effects of oestrogen helping balance levels required for satisfying sex.

Persistent Genital Arousal Disorder
This is more a male affliction, where the poor man is permanently on the edge of climax. It is embarrassing and painful and orgasm does not assuage his symptoms.

Perhaps marjoram, with its anaphrodisiac medicine (puts you off sex) might help or maybe yarrow to calm the pain.

Impotence
That's probably a whole book on its own but hopefully the recommendations in the next chapter can help to remove any emotional issues. Jasmine helps create a harder erection. Erections are controlled by nitric oxide, a gas neurotransmitter which rushes through the tissues. Clove is proven to affect nitric oxide levels. However, I think, topically might do little else than create a burning sensation, unless you use in dilutions of less than 0.25% on such a sensitive area. Nutmeg too, is a support to the pituitary gland responsible for the formation of sexual hormones.

Diffusion is a very good idea rather than topically warming to eyewatering levels with nutmeg and clove! You'll affect the neurotransmitters and create an atmosphere of Christmas cosiness.

Orgasm

Sexual Differences of Climax

Women climax for longer, but men get off more often. A man will take around four minutes of stimulation whereas women usually require between 10-20 minutes, although there have been reported studies of ladies who can come with just thirty seconds of masturbation. A woman's climax averages 20 seconds, a man's orgasm averages just three. Blokes have ejaculatory threshold, the so-called "point of no return" requiring a certain amount of stimulation to bring him to climax. Women, do not have this, and take longer, and can even lose an orgasm right in the middle. Interestingly, studies show that a woman needs to feel deeply relaxed and very safe, with no sense of anxiety to experience orgasm. Likewise, she is less likely to climax if she feels insecure about her relationship.

The belief that women can climax many times and men can only come once is a myth, with men physiologically able to orgasm both before and after their semen release. Indeed, the first documented evidence of an awareness of men multiply orgasming dates back to Chinese papers from 2968 B.C.

The most documented orgasms in one hour is 134 for women and just 6 for a man.

Surveys show 95% men climax during sex, but only 69 % of women manage to. Lesbians are 12% more likely to than straight women, but scientists suggest this is probably more down to the type of sex they are having rather than a sexual difference. It can probably be put down to the length of time they are enjoying sex, 10-15 mins intercourse for straight women as opposed to half an hour if you are gay.

Scientists relate that men and women both use the same kinds of words to describe their orgasms leading them to suspect that feel similar. This might be because penile and clitoral tissues are identical, since foetuses share female genitalia during the first trimester of growth. It's only when boys begin to secrete testosterone at around 12 weeks that the tissue forms into male genitalia.

Regardless of differences, the physiological effects of orgasm are the same for all. Both sexes go through the same four stages of arousal: excitement, plateau, orgasm, and resolution.

Brain stimulation increases heart rate and blood flow speeds to the genitals. During climax, brain scans show massive changes in waves across all areas. Interestingly the activity is not restricted to the areas of physical gratification but also lights up the emotional and spiritual areas of the brain too. We might recognise the sensations of the logical areas of the mind shutting down, (the orbitofrontal cortex controlling how we evaluate ourselves and reason) as the sensation of losing ourselves *into le petit mort.*

During climax, the body is flooded with the ecstasy hormone prolactin which then makes us snoozy and want to curl up and go to sleep.

Women and Orgasm
It is thought that only around two thirds of women easily experience orgasm, and just 80% of those reach climax through

vaginal intercourse. Recent research suggests your ability to climax maybe genetic and it is thought the distance between a woman's vagina and her clitoris directly relates to how easily she can come. The closer it is, the more stimulation it receives. Doctors all seem to agree that pelvic floor exercises (Kegels) increase the likelihood of women getting off.

Not all girls need their downstairs bits rubbing. Some climax by nipple stimulation alone, which makes sense, because scans show the nipple and vagina stimulation zones are the same parts of the brain. Many ladies come from kissing alone and some just by thinking about coming! About 5% are believed to have "coregasms" from exercise and some can even climax during childbirth. A very, very rare number orgasm from sneezing. I wonder how many handkerchiefs they need to carry in their bags?

For most though, clitoral stimulation is the best possible avenue to bliss, with the organ being equipped with no less than 8000 nerve endings. However, depending on how you were stimulated to orgasm will dictate how it feels, because different nerves connect the various erogenous zones to the brain. That gasp of electric you feel shoot up your spine when you are touched is your pudendal nerve connecting the clitoris (and his penis) to the brain. A vaginal orgasm feels deeper, communicated through the pelvic nerves. The cervix is connected to the brain via the hypogastric, pelvic and vagus nerves which all transmit feelings of pleasure via different routes. Therefore, it is possible to create a deeper and more intense orgasm by stimulation of two or more erogenous zones simultaneously, sending pleasure rippling through several areas of the body.

Orgasms also differ depending on what time of your menstrual cycle you have them. Most of the month the pelvic muscles roll inward into the body, but during your period, the muscles open outward and open, presuably to push invading debris and invaders out of the body.

For a small number of women, orgasm can be horrifyingly embarrassing as they gush liquid in female ejaculation. The most moving account of this must surely be found in Eve Ensler's play "The Vagina Monologues" where one woman described "The Flood" after being kissed ardently in a dishy young man's car. He'd been cruel and called her "weird stink girl", and took her home, in silence, furious at her for soiling her car. Later she describes how she had nightmares throughout her life about being caught off guard by passion, and even how eventually, the doctor seemed whimsical about removing her "downstairs bits" when she developed cancer, saying "If you don't use it, you lose it". The incident had deeply affected her life and when asked what her vagina would say if it could talk, she answered "Closed due to flooding".

Scientists are still unsure what this liquid is and whether it serves any adaptation function in the process. Many women worry they have wet the bed, and indeed ultrasounds show that some women's bladders speedily fill and empty during climax. However, the fluid contains no urea and is colourless, not staining the sheets.

Other women secrete a thick white milky substance from the urethra, which is very similar in nature to semen, but without the sperm. It is thought it is released from the skene glands, structures akin to the prostate gland in men. A third type of female ejaculation seems to be a mix of the two, where scientists have analysed the fluid lost (usually about half a coffee cupful) and have found it contains traces of this white fluid.

Contrary to what the porn and erotica industry would have us believe, only a small number of women ejaculate, although it does seem likely that the ejaculation may be related to stimulation of the g-spot, a small section of tissue at the front of the vagina that increases pleasure enormously. Luckily, not all men find it as abhorrent as the boy in the car, and many think it testament to their manhood and find it all the more attractive.

Perhaps presumed to be a modern trend, Aristotle was the first to describe female ejaculation and Galen also wrote of it in the 2nd Century AD. That said, it has recently become somewhat taboo. Scenes with female ejaculation have now been banned from British porn films as being obscene. (Although I have to say any decision that talks about women's physiology like that, seems far obscener than any graphic on the screen!) However, perhaps this will bring an end to the pressure of the media, that all women should be "gushing", when actually it is a very small proportion of women who do, and even those capable, perhaps only experience it once in their life.

Where men experience wet dreams, about 37% of women admit to having had at least one orgasm when they have been asleep

Studies of interviews with women, seem to suggest that partners don't give women an orgasm, they consciously or unconsciously allow themselves to climax. Anxiety, poor self-image, distrust, feeling betrayed or distracting thoughts are all enough to switch her brain off and end the climax.

Men and Orgasm

It is possible to orgasm without ejaculating and the ancient technique of Tantra trains men to do this through command of a technique called fire breathing. Usually, he will have a "retrograde period" of around 30 minutes to recover after climax but it is possible for men to have many orgasms one after another.

Research shows that orgasms may protect your man from cancer, with men who have more than twenty a month having a lower risk of prostate cancer (Twenty?!) It's thought the benefit probably comes from the release of oxytocin that also reduces blood pressure.

Contrary to the belief that only women fake, a 2010 study of college students showed that 25% of men had faked an orgasm some time in their lives.

Ejaculation is fast...no I mean *really* fast. Usain Bolt runs at 29.79 mph and semen shoots out at 28mph. Interestingly, the swimmers at the front of the queue are also proven to be the sperm with the best DNA.

Orgasm and Pain

Orgasm has clearly defined benefits to health including a direct relationship between regular orgasms and better immune systems. However, it is also quintessentially linked to the reduction of pain. In brain scans, the anterior cingulate cortex and the insula both light up during climax, areas usually associated with pain. Potentially this might be why we look like we are in agony as we experience such pleasure.

More though, a woman experiences as radical reduction in pain during and after climax, 107% in total, lasting for between 1-8 minutes afterwards.

Pain Disorders

I don't think I will be saying too much about my sex life to say I have suffered one of these for twenty years. To my own mind I think it might be related to a combination of a very violent ex-partner and a traumatic incident while giving birth. Certainly, there are times when it is better and times when it is worse, usually related to my menstrual cycle and also to times of stress.

I have found essential oils a great help in relaxing me enough to enjoy the experience. Oils such as clary sage and yarrow prevent me from tensing up and yuzu keeps my mind from worrying about when the pain will strike. By far the best though is a marijuana blend into coconut oil, where the THC gets my bits too high to care!!!! (Both good girl and naughty mix versions are in the recipes section of the cannabis book.)

Since there are a distressingly wide number of these pain disorders, I'm not going to describe them all, except to say many have their roots in emotional issues, so oils can help from that dimension. If you are not clear what is causing yours, I would start by experimenting with oils that:

Relax Muscles:

Juniper, Lavender, Sweet Basil, Clary Sage, Black Pepper, Ginger, Roman Chamomile, Geranium, Yarrow, Myrrh

Relax Connective Tissue

Frankincense, Clary Sage

Relax Nerves

Rosemary, Peppermint, Roman Chamomile, Cistus, Clary Sage, Catnip, Rose, Sandalwood, Vetiver, Neroli & Ylang Ylang

Antispasmodic

Clary Sage, Angelica (Root & Seed), Cardamom, Caraway, Black Spruce, Palo Santo, Vetiver, Spikenard, Yarrow, Rose

Chapter 2 Stress and Its Effects on Sex

I'm going to begin by saying if you are stressed, anxious, depressed, in pain or struggling with infertility...then you should be taking High CBD Hemp Oil.

Cannabidiol interacts with the endocannabinoid system (eCS) to ensure levels of hormones and neurotransmitters stay correct. If libido has dropped, fertility isn't happening, or you are experiencing pain during sex, CBD is where I would start. Sort out those hormone levels and get that neurochemical balance right. No matter what essential oils you use, if the eCS is fighting against you, it is going to be like an elastic band that keeps snapping back. A very big subject, far too big for this book, read 400 pages of data about it in my cannabis book.

Hormone Levels

When we are stressed or afraid, the HPA axis kicks in. This mechanism of the **H**ypothalamus, **P**ituitary, and **A**drenals involves the hypothalamus triggering CRF (Corticotrophin Releasing Factor) to be released from the pituitary and then ACTH (adrenocorticotrophic hormone) from the adrenals.

Cortisol is made from ACTH. Short term, cortisol is healthy working as an anti-inflammatory for the body, but after a while it will change to becoming inflammatory attacking the heart and other organs in the body.

During periods of long terms stress, the adrenals continue to secrete hormones, but eventually will tire and begin to look for other sources of energy. First port of call is the liver, creating many stress related responses and then the adrenals act like parasites to the pituitary.

The pituitary secretes many hormones, many of them related to reproduction. They stimulate ovulation, ripen eggs, and stimulate labour and milk when baby has been born. In men, these hormones trigger the testes to manufacture testosterone and sperm too.

Stress directly influences many neurotransmitters, relevantly to sex: dopamine, serotonin, and oxytocin.

The Neurochemistry of Sex

Dopamine

Dopamine dictates whether we will want sex or not. Correct levels keep us motivated, satisfied, trusting and open with people, taking calculated risks with realistic expectations, and capable of loving as a parent.

In excess, we will see sexual fetishes, perversions and addictions, risk-taking, compulsive and addictive behaviour, aggression and in some cases anxiety. Worse, schizophrenia and psychosis both have their roots firmly planted in skewed dopamine levels, Deficiency leaves us with little interest in life, no pursuit of pleasure and depression. Often low levels will lead to loss of libido and impotence, there is an inability to love with no remorse for bad behaviour. Social Anxiety Disorder and anti-social behaviour are both associated with low levels of dopamine.

So, we can see immediately how dopamine is going to be our first hurdle.

Oils Proven to Affect Dopamine Levels Are:

Lemon, Clary Sage, Cedarwood, Eucalyptus, Blue Lotus & Orange.

Serotonin

This is our mood modulator which has a direct bearing of whether we are literally "In the mood". Serotonin's part in sex is less understood and seems to be more involved with social interaction rather than sex per se.

However, when scientists engineered rats without serotonin, they made some very peculiar findings. They expected to find they had created gay mice (I will confess to not having a clue why they thought that!) but something rather different took place. Instead, these rats were hypersexual, completely indiscriminate of whether they humped males or females. It looks like levels of serotonin probably influence hypo- or hyper-sexuality. On the surface, this currently looks like levels may make you sexually indiscriminate, but since so many receptors appear in such a variety of areas of the brain, it is still not understood if that is true, why that might be, or whether there is indeed more going on.

Physiologically, during sex, scientists suspect it is the strange interplay between epinephrine and serotonin that creates the delicious pulsating sensation in the genitals. Serotonin constricts and epinephrine fights to soften the tissues, serotonin constricts it again.

Oils for Serotonin Levels

Most relaxing and uplifting top notes are going to influence serotonin, really. Think lemon, orange, bergamot and melissa to level out parameters and support healthy libido.

So, throughout sex the Central Nervous System sends messages to the heart, imploring it to pump faster, sending oxygenated blood to the muscles used in sexual activity. As the blood starts to race, neurotransmitters all dance together creating a symphony of ecstatic union.

Nitric oxide catapults through the cells, releasing smooth muscle and increasing blood flow to the penis. Serotonin constricts the smooth muscles and nerves of the genitals. Epinephrine constantly fights to keep the penis flaccid and increases the force and rate of its contraction. A woman experiences epinephrine's embrace as it increases the amplitude of her vaginal pulse. Every moment you become more aroused, epinephrine pumps more.

Prolactin
Later, after orgasm dies, nature's conspiracy in the battle of the sexes continues. If any of you have read Men are From Mars, Women from Venus, you will recognise John Gray's description of men needing to emotionally withdraw after sex and for a few days he "disappears into his cave".

I wonder if the explanation for that might come from differences in neurotransmission.

Dopamine falls rapidly after orgasm plummeting immediately in men, but reducing more slowly in women taking longer to begin to fall. In its place, prolactin floods the body. It has been circulating for a while as what we have felt as ecstasy, but then lingers in the tissues for longer.

Prolactin brings about a lack of libido, explaining the male's refractory period of no more sex for a while. It makes him impotent and sends us all to sleep. It brings about mood changes and depression, making women anxious and hostile. Weirdly, an excess of prolactin can create menopausal symptoms in women even when she has perfectly adequate levels of oestrogen. Excess also causes weight gain and vaginal dryness.

The physiological intention of prolactin is to give a fertilised egg the very best chance it has for survival, chasing any other suitors away. Amazingly, it takes two weeks for levels of prolactin to completely subside, explaining why many people find their partners thoroughly irritating for several days after sex.

Essential Oils That Influence Prolactin

Chasteberry essential oil *(Vitus agnus castus) is* proven to affect levels of prolactin and may also help women whose prolactin levels have created a testosterone rich environment. Signs of this might include excess body hair and Poly Cystic Ovarian Syndrome. Isn't the name Chasteberry adorable in this context? How gifted were our ancients?!

So, Nature then looked at The Humans and shook Her head, not trusting that we would not rip each other apart swimming in in an ocean of prolactin. She worried who would look after this possible created child. Smiling, She created oxytocin.

Oxytocin
The cuddling hormone, a neuropeptide formed in the hypothalamus.

It seems likely that oxytocin and dopamine are inextricably linked. Together they regulate tissues in an erection, and oxytocin seems to express dopamine receptors. Nature partnered oxytocin with prolactin to ensure that, despite the fact we want to smash each other's faces in sometimes, this molecule makes us want to stay together.

It is also the yin to cortisol's yang. Where cortisol is manufactured through fear, oxytocin is born out of love. Cortisol arouses us, stresses us out makes us feel anxious and aggressive, and is associated with depression; oxytocin calms us and makes us feel more connected. It increases curiosity and increases sexual receptivity, cortisol by contrast lowers libido.

Cortisol activates addictions (through its dopamine interaction) where oxytocin *lessens* cravings and addition.

Cortisol weakens the immune system; breaks down bones muscular, and connective tissues; it clogs arteries, promotes heart disease, high blood pressure, obesity, diabetes, and osteoporosis and increases pain. Oxytocin diminishes the sense of pain, lowers blood pressure, protects against heart disease, and brings about faster wound healing.

In addition, the love hormone, released through nipple stimulation and orgasm facilitates learning, heals, repairs, and restores our body. It bonds a couple together, facilitates birth and brings in the milk when a baby is born.

Oddly though, and far be it from me to question Her genius, but men aren't anywhere near as affected by the oxytocin as women since high levels of testosterone seem to drown out oxytocin's song. So, where women are falling deeper and deeper in love with him, it takes several songs for him to hear it. That's possibly why men create ties much more slowly and view those first few initial contacts as just sex. That said research shows that the oxytocin levels stay higher and have a better chance of levelling out the dopamine rollercoaster if closer proximity is maintained for a while after sex.

Interestingly, in studies where men were shown pictures of the opposite sex, men found pictures of their own partner the most attractive of the group, when levels of oxytocin were high. Levels are found to be naturally higher in couples who display non-verbal expressive displays of affection. Higher levels are also related to feelings of love, satisfaction with the relationship and more feelings of gratitude.

Oils Encouraging Oxytocin Levels Are:

Celery Seed, Cinnamon, Fennel, Black Cumin Seed And Evening Primrose Carrier Oil.

You might want to create a diffuser oil for later, since the prolactin will put paid to wanting to massage and hopefully your knees will be too wobbly to get out of bed.

Trying to Get Pregnant
Essential oils help fertility but the second you think you might be pregnant you need to stop using topically. To be clear, there has never been a proven reported case of miscarriage explicitly caused by essential oils, but since we don't know how they affect forming foetuses, I believe it is better to avoid oils and give your pregnancy the very best chance it can have.

This stopping and starting is a complicated and stressful dance so I usually advice people take a six month break from trying and just use essential oils to boost fertility levels, tone the uterus, calm stress and enjoy some great pressure free sex. When the time is over, and the charts come back out, switch to diffusion only and refrain from topical use for a while.

Oils to Boost Fertility Are:

Rose, Clary Sage, Jasmine, Geranium, Ylang Ylang & Nutmeg.

Chapter 3 – Has Anyone Seen Where I Left My Sensuality?

I can't speak for men, but as a woman, I think most of us lose touch with sensuality somewhere between washing up and taking the kids to school. It's incredibly easy to get so caught up in the rush of "Have to..." we forget to take a moment to enjoy the "want to" in life.

And, as time ticks away, we become further detached from our physical body and soon there is a disconnect. We feel completely dissected from our sensual selves. It's no wonder most of us can't really be bothered to have sex! The joyful news is, that sensuality does remain, albeit a bit dusty, and can be reignited with a little coaxing.

Stimulating our sense of smell, perfume, of course, plays a part, but there is more. Take time to focus on the tastes you are putting into your mouth, deeply experience nuances of sweetness, bitterness and sour. Perhaps set aside five minutes a day to just taste, smell, touch, and listen to beautiful music.

I can't recommend dancing enough to you. Dance like no-one is watching and ramp the stereo up full blast; belt your favourite songs out at the top of your lungs. Bend, slide, get those legs open, slide your hands over your body, stroke the vortices of chakric energy, pushing the vital energy of kundalini upwards from the pelvis right up to the crown. Loose yourself in the music and be completely you.

See yourself. Start looking at yourself in the mirror. Get intimate with how you look with no clothes on. Take a few moments to consider what is truly unique and fantastic about your body. Do you have lovely eyes, cracking boobs, a booty Beyoncé would be proud of? Find something and really focus on it.

Sophia Loren once said: "Sex appeal is 50% what you've got and 50% what people think you've got!" Stand up straight. Get those shoulders back, show off that bust, walk with confidence and sass.

Luxuriate in warm candlelit bubble baths and stroke rich luxurious creams and lotions into your skin.

Start a love affair with yourself, because at times when compliments are not forthcoming, you need someone reliable to remind you how great you are. Think of ten things that are truly amazing about you and keep telling yourself every day why you damn well rock!

Smile at yourself and say –

"I am sexy and beautiful."

•I am a vixen, a sensual, sexual woman.

•I embrace my womanhood, my body, and my sexuality.

•I open myself up to receiving as well as giving pleasure.

Fake confidence until it comes true, (and it will) because I promise you there is nothing sexier than feeling and looking like you feel amazing.

Desire

In our Western culture we all seem to   be searching for that elusive "chemistry", that mystical spark that sets us alight. This is a very modern point of view and ancient societies all placed far more emphasis on the creation of good sex than something that mystically appeared.

The Kama Sutra is a famous sexual manual that dates to the 2nd Century BC. Famous for its erotic graphical deigns of sexual positions, a far greater portion of the book is given over to the mastery of creation of beauty, as part of desire. Rather than our perfunctory sex, with the light off on Friday night, ancient Indian, Chinese, and Japanese traditions all put far more emphasis on sexual partnership as ritual. And while that may seem a bit contrived in today's day and age, it ensured that effort, beauty, and tenderness were all part of the seduction process too.

Incidentally, the name "Kama" means "erotic practice" and "Sutra" means "holds life together."

One area of the masterpiece relates how a room was set aside away from the rest of the house, furnished only with a bed, flowers and incense and a bathroom. Its sole purpose was marital seduction. How lovely would it be to recreate that mystery again?

The instructions explain how the gentleman bathes dresses in his finest clothing. Ceremonially ready, he invites friends and servants to come and join him in the "Chamber of Love."

He seats himself beside his woman, brings her something enticing to drink and eloquently chatters to her about *stuff,* riddles, gossip. Very gradually, he slowly adds more risqué themes to arouse her.

Phase two of seduction begins as music and song engage the room and, suggests the Kama Sutra the couple might feel they would like to get up and dance. Later, they discuss art and our hero encourages his lady to take another drink.

Chatting softly to her, staring into her eyes, gently, he strokes her hair. Slightly woozy, perhaps distracted she may not notice as he loosens her robe in the area between her thighs. Perhaps he might show her phallic drawings in to excite her more.

Eventually he scents her with floral essences and serves her aphrodisiac betel leaves, a cue for guests to leave our lovers alone together in the Chamber of Love. Ardently he "tears off her robe" and makes love to her using positions chosen to give her most pleasure, taking into consideration their body types and sizes of their sexual organs.

Afterwards, they retire to the bathroom, taking separate quarters to clean up before returning to their bed.

Gently he tends to any bumps or bruises she may have sustained rubbing sandalwood paste all over her body. Wrapping his arms about her he whispers sweetly in her ear while gently feedsing her *"grilled meats, drinks of ripe fruit juice... then, at their ease, they drink sweet liquor, while chewing from time to time sweet or tart things."*

Later, climbing up to the roof terrace to bask in the moonlight, they continue to talk through the night.

It's shocking to see how different sex was then to how it is today. Frankly, I like their way better! But is it always the man who must be instigator?

The Courtesan
The feminist in me could not leave this book without mentioning the ancient role of courtesan, now vilified in today's society, and somehow relegated to role of whore.

Not so. Mistress, yes. But prostitute sells her short.

In Ancient societies such as the Greeks, this mistress of the bedroom enjoyed the same societal privileges as men while wives were locked away at home. Often, they had their own houses complete with servants, and sometimes took in other women to look after them and coax them in their art.

But their skills were not only limited to sex; in fact, far from it. These were powerful and intelligent women; their brains rich with intellect and wit. The kama sutra tells us these women should be proficient in no less than 64 subjects from cooking and painting, to woodwork. These women were enjoyed, but also enjoyed themselves, having made a conscious decision to exchange sex for the freedom to engage and further their minds. A man might take his courtesan for life but should not, society dictated, marry her.

The courtesan knew how to make a man feel special. For those few short hours he was centre of her world. He had invested time and money in honing her courtship and sexual techniques exploring new positions and even using toys. For his arrival, she would always be dressed alluringly and ready for the triste. In return threw money and worship in her direction in the hope of keeping her interested, because at the sniff of a better deal, the courtesan was off. Sorry, Mister, that exclusivity was over.

Today, marriage doesn't (shouldn't) have the same restraints. Women are free to continue their education and climb career ladders, but I do think there is now a role for courtesan inside of a marriage. Engaging your partners mind is every bit as important as their loins! One might go so far as to say the sexiest organ might just be the brain.

We all know couples who live together but live out their passion outside the home. Their greatest attention is their job, the hairdressers, the gym or the golf course, and there just isn't space in that relationship for a lover. If this describes you, then perhaps it is time to learn how to court.

Chapter 4 The Oils That Turn the Science into An Art

Thus far, we have talked science, about how oils can help on the most physical levels, easing muscles and nerves, relaxing us and balancing neurotransmission. That's the easy bit. Even the doctor can get that far with his pills and lotions. ☐

Now we start aromatherapy. This where the good bit begins, and I must say thank you to one of my readers Jeanne Butcher who suggested the title should be *50 places ylang and ylang and patchouli can't reach*, which is bang on (no pun intended!) and Sarah Cooper who made me giggle with *"Things that are stinky and kinky."* Clever gals, you both!

But this is where we say...What can we do about how you feel? How can we undo the guilt you feel about wanting sex when your religion says you shouldn't? How can we let go of the feelings of betrayal and start again? How do we leave the negative associations of the past and have a hopeful start with a new love?

Essential oils? You know it.

Potentially for as many feelings that we might have, I suspect there are even more essential oils. Probably ones we can't find in the shops because they don't smell great, are hazardous or even protected as a species. No matter. We have ample here. But know these are my thoughts and interactions with the oils. Yours may be different and just as your history may create negative associations with places, songs or foods, so does your mind with fragrances too. Experiment together.

Amber

Pinus Succinifera

Not strictly an essential oil (good start isn't it!) this is an oil infusion of fossilized resins from an amalgamation of many different resin trees.

Amber must be 35, 000 years old to own its name, so, there is something incredibly steadfast about amber. There is a longevity to it and a deep sense of what went before. I use amber for lifting trauma (along with cistus / labdanum). It has a deep resonating base note that acts as the perfect fixative for blends where sensuality is no-existent because of some kind of deep seated emotional injury. Blend with frankincense to connect with the psyche and help the body begin the healing process together. Blend with myrrh to instil trust.

Blending Note: Base

Character: Earthy, Golden Balsamic, Vaguely Pine Fragranced

Blends Well With:

Top Notes:

Lemon Verbena, Lemon Grass, Lemon, Mandarin, Tangerine, Orange, Petitgrain

Heart Notes:

Rose, Geranium, Palmarosa, Frankincense

Base Notes:

Sandalwood, Myrrh, Agarwood.

Maximum Dilution 3%

Cautions: Not suitable for use during the first 16 weeks of pregnancy.

Amyris
Amyris balsamifera

Amyris is often confused with Sandalwood but, in my opinion doesn't have the orgasmic appeal of the real oil. That, being said, it is a wonderful oil for repairing arguments and encouraging a spirit of openness and receptivity.

Easing muscle spasms and restlessness, it calms restlessness and allows you to sink into relaxation.

Blending Note: Base

Character: Soothing, Meditative, Slowing, Opening, Peaceful & Balsamic

Top Notes: Citronella, Orange, Melissa, Lemongrass

Heart Notes: Ylang Ylang, Ginger, Ho Wood, Lavender,

Base Notes: Peru balsam and Cedarwood

Maximum Dilution: 3%

Cautions: *Not suitable for topical use during first 16 weeks of pregnancy*

Agarwood
Aquilaria malaccensis

A controversial oil, I often try to weave it into essays for professional journals but then get asked to remove it because it is a protected species. I agree, however I only source mine from sustainable resources and I thought I would take the opportunity to introduce you to something truly erotic (as well as being wonderful for stress, cardiac and respiratory conditions.)

This precious oil is taken from the heartwood of the *Aquilaria malaccensis* tree, but the dark wood only manifests essence when damaged, sometimes by a parasite, sometimes by lightening etc. Often affected trees can be very old, and felling them to find it, means there will be no oil contained within.

The precious oil, also sometimes known as Oudh, smells so incredible that, sadly it was almost felled to extinction. Thus, it has been placed under protected measures. Earlier this millennium, scientists discovered it was possible to irritate young trees into production by injecting it with herbal oils and a brand-new world of oil production has been born.

The oil I use is from trees grown in Malaysia from sustainable crops. Oil can be extracted when the tree is around ten years old and trees are then replaced for ongoing growth and production.

Its fragrance is like nothing like any I can think of. It is deep, thick and sultry, almost balsamic, vanilla chocolate qualities. Extremely masculine, with an animalic, leathery fragrance reminiscent of autumnal rotting wood, it is rich, profound and lingers for hours and hours. I promise you, any blends with this in it will still be reminding you of the previous night's passion for most of the next day!

Agarwood, or sometimes known as Aloeswood seems to come from a different world to the mine. It transports me out of the serenity of the English countryside into the richness of Scheherazade, Eastern souks, temples, hareems and magic carpets! Gorgeous.

Blending Note: Basest of The Base Notes!

Character: Masculine in Nature. Soothing, Reflective & Mesmeric.

Blends Well With:

Top Note: Lemon, Lemon Grass, Lemon Verbena, Mandarin, Melissa, Orange, Petitgrain, Yuzu

Heart Note Florals, Spices & Evergreen Trees!

Rose, Jasmine, Spikenard, Ambrette Seed, Juniper, Fir Ginger,

Base Note: Woods, Resins & Spikenard!

Amber, Amyris, Frankincense, Labdanum, Sandalwood,

Benzoin
Benzoin styrax

This is not directly an aphrodisiac oil as such, but is warming, comforting, and relaxing. Somehow it seems to bring energy to the sexual organs flooding them with stronger circulation, invigorating and releasing them.

It is euphoric, clearing and emptying the conscious mind. Seemingly, it moves the heart away from the hustle and bustle of the outside world, into the very quietest of places, nurturing and allowing tensions to just drift away. A lovely oil to remove distracting thoughts and to leave stress behind for a few short hours.

Benzoin is the perfect link to tone super sweet oils, lending a soft, smoothness to them

Blending Note: Base

Character: Resinous, Medicinal. Comforting, Reassuring, Silky Soft & Balancing.

Blends Well With:

Top Notes: All Citruses & Sweet Notes

Heart Notes: Sweet Notes Like Rose, Geranium & Ylang Ylang. Pungent Spices Like Black Pepper

Base Notes: Myrrh, Galbanum, Sandalwood

Maximum Dilution - 3%

Cautions: *Not suitable for topical use during first 16 weeks of pregnancy*

Bergamot
Citrus bergamia

Not strictly aphrodisiac, but bergamot brings out playful mischief in other oils that are! Where jasmine or ylang ylang are languorous, stretching out like a cat, bergamot is enticing and frolicsome, lifting your emotions and bringing a smile to your face. Bergamot is a naughty wink that says come on then, I dare ya!

Beguiling and antidepressant, bergamot eases the day away and over time can be a potent emotional healer, lending support in the darkest of moments. If sensuality is buried in gloom, then gentle touch with bergamot can often be the light at the end of the tunnel.

Since no-one wants a snoozefest after putting so much work into seduction, there is certainly plenty of good things to say about an oil that wakes you up too!

But, for all its friskiness, bergamot is refined, elegant and quintessentially ladylike. She adds class to the occasion, preventing sultry tawdriness. Sophisticated panache, with a hint of giggles.

Blending Note: Bright, Vivacious, Giggly Top Note.

Character: Feminine, Wily, Flirtatious & Giggly.

Blends well with: *Almost everything, she is a popular lass who gets on well with everyone.*

Top Note: Lemon, Lemon Grass, Lemon Verbena, Mandarin, Melissa, Orange, Petitgrain, Yuzu, Cinnamon, Black Pepper, Nutmeg

Heart Note Florals, Herbs, and Evergreen Trees!

Lavender, Rose, Geranium & Jasmine, Basil, Rosemary, Coriander, Spikenard, Ambrette Seed, Juniper, Fir & Ginger.

Base Note: Amber, Amyris, Cedarwood, Frankincense, Labdanum, Myrrh, Sandalwood & Spikenard

Safety: Safe only after 16 weeks of pregnancy.

Bergamot is expressed from the peel of the fruit and like many other oils extracted this way, can be phototoxic. Do not expose the skin to sunlight (or sunbeds!) for 12 hours after use. Do not use old oils. High levels of monoterpenes which can decay very quickly causing risk of skin sensitisation.

Blue Lotus
Nymphaea Caerulea

The first time I heard of this oil was when Roxanne Benton on Aromamatrix told me a story of a lady who had smelt some on the stand and got a little on her hands. She'd gone to the toilet, clearly inadvertently transferred it to a sensitive area and re-arrived at the stand looking sated, flushed and declaring "I haven't had an experience like that in years!"

Well, it had my attention!

It is a mild psychedelic when added to wine, is euphoric, and a potent aphrodisiac. *Nymphaea caerulea* is native to Egypt. Mentioned in the ancient Egyptian *Book of The Dead*, it was a ritual plant for both the living and those despatched to the afterlife. Almost every temple is decorated with the lotus image, pillars, walls, and tombs are all adorned alike. Oddly though, nowadays, the lotus is seldom found growing naturally in Egypt.

Modern day Egyptians still revere the lotus as the primordial symbol of creation and rebirth, only appearing above the water for three days then plummeting back to the gloom depths for another year.

Ancient sacraments were created by priests and pharaohs, steeping the flowers for many days to create a connection of consciousness to commune with the sun-god Ra. Some scholars believe the sacrament might also have been taken at rituals of the goddess of love and fertility, Isis.

It's driving action of promoting desire probably comes from the constituent apomorphine, a dopamine agonist, which could (I suspect) lead to addiction issues if not used with care.

Lotus is warming and lightning, there is an unmistakable feeling of lightness around the head, when you use it. It is dreamy and incredibly relaxing.

Apart from the obvious advantages of such an overtly aphrodisiac oil, it is antispasmodic and wonderful for pelvic pain. It loosens and unwinds the pelvis, opening and softening it making it more available for people with problems with vaginal tenderness or pelvic pain to enjoy sex less painfully. This pelvic action also extends to alleviate menstrual pain or tenderness after caesarean.

Blue Lotus is a sacrament of worship, so it's not really an oil for casual sex. It is desire encapsulated in love, wholeness and union. Incredibly helpful to relationships that have lost that loving edge and a chasm is beginning to open between them. Connecting lovers to the divine sacrament and isolating them from external disturbances, it centres them on the precipice of a joint pedestal.

Blending Note: Top to Middle

Character: Intense, Hypnotic, Beguiling, Other-Worldly, Energetic, Consuming & Vivid

Blends well with:

Top Note: Citrus & Spicy

Lime, Neroli, Bergamot
Heart Note Florals, Herbs & Evergreen Trees!
Rose, Geranium, Basil, Rosemary, Cumin, Spikenard, Juniper, Fir & Ginger,
Base Note: Myrrh, Agarwood & Sandalwood

Maximum Dilution: 3%

Safety: Not suitable during pregnancy.

Cardamom
Elletaria Cardomomum

One of the key ingredients in Eastern traditions, cardamom is a spice of seduction. Often added to coffee at varying times of preparation, Bedouins place cardamom pods into the spout of the coffee pot to ensure just the right amount of fragrance to each cup!

It eases the flow of conversation, making your words silky sweet, weaving a spell of enchantment around those who hear you. It prevents second guessing, liberating bedrooms from the worries of "Will this happen?" It allows a person to just be, relaxing the mind into the present. There is something very sturdy about cardamom; it instils emotional stamina. If a problem is taking a long time to repair, it instils patience but also hope and motivation for the future.

Ruled by Venus, she imbues love, but also the gentleness and warmth of Mars. This is empowered and equal loving, independence, and a relationship on clearly defined and equal terms. Perfect union.

Cardamom enhances libido, breaks down emotional barriers and dissipates the tensions of frigidity.

Blending Note: Heart

Character: Spicy-Sweet, Nutty, Woody, Vaguely Aniseed-Y, Welcoming & Releasing.

Blends Well With:

Top Notes: Orange, Lemon, Palmarosa & Citronella

Heart Notes: Cinnamon, Caraway, Cloves &Ginger

Base Notes: Vetiver, Agarwood & Myrrh

Maximum Dilution 3%

Cautions: *Not suitable for use in the first 16 weeks of pregnancy.*

Catnip
Nepeta cataria

I must tell you a story unrelated to sex, because I can't use catnip without thinking of it. My friend Alan Howell of Sechina Essential Oils once told me the largest ever order he took, was for a massive quantity of catnip from a zoo who were going to have to put a tiger to sleep. They wanted it to have the most blissful and submissive ending it could. Isn't that beautiful?!

Many of us will be familiar of how batty cats go around catnip, and to a certain extent humans are the same and it is a herb that appears over and over in love spells. It is reputed to make women more attractive and to make men ready. More, it has strong associations with the love and fertility goddesses Sekhmet and Bast (not surprising really, I suppose, a cat goddess) and is said to help barren women if they drink the leaves in a tea. Just as cats go daft, so there is a playfulness about catnip; it is gentle and light hearted. It is a wonderful pick me up if you feel sluggish and lethargic.

For those of you who would like to entice a new lover, apparently carrying a bag of catnip with you will entice the man you desire, and making a concoction of catnip, cinnamon of rum will help you too. Witches tell me you should sprinkle it for 21 days outside your front door and then wait for love to come knocking. (Please do tell me if you do this and it works!)

If you suspect your sexuality may have been affected by anxiety, then this is the oil for you. Specifically, it is helpful for people who worry and then internalise the anxiety into the physical body. It is a strong antispasmodic, relieving both cramping but also menstrual pains.

Blending Note: Top

Character: Playful, Narcotic, Silly, Whimsical, Relaxing & Unorthodox

Top Note: Lemon, Lime, Peppermint, Grapefruit & Orange

Heart Note: Eucalyptus, Lavender, Lavandin, Marjoram & Rosemary

Base Note: Myrrh

Cedarwood Atlas
Cedrus atlantica

In amongst all these flowers and feminine oils there exists a truly stead-fast male, cedarwood. It is soothing and calming, easing the mind away from worries and releasing it from the shackles from obsessive thinking. Bursting with sesquiterpenes, it pacifies the brain, absorbing you into a peaceful embrace.

Since time immemorial, ancient civilisations have revered the cedars of Lebanon for their long straight and sturdy trunks, creating great temples with one of the only woods they would trust to connect them to the divine. Incenses and embalming fluids alike, took priests and Pharaohs on godlike journeys to connect with a higher source. Emptying their minds of the everyday, they were transported to a quieter place of reflection. Cedarwood holds you tight. It smothers away concerns and immerses you in the present. Nothing else matters except for here.

Blending Note: Base

Character: Woody, Meditative, Soothing, Grounding, Absorbent, Distancing & Immersive.

Blends Well With:

Top Notes: Bergamot, Cajuput, Lemon & Other Citruses, Cinnamon, Petitgrain & Neroli

Heart Notes: Spices, Herbaceous Notes & Florals

Base Notes: Sandalwood, Myrrh & Spikenard

Maximum Dilution: 3%

Cautions: *Not suitable for topical use during first 16 weeks of pregnancy*

Celery Seed

Few people seem to write much about celery seed, but I think it is an incredibly powerful oil. Mentally and spiritually cleansing, it allows you to focus. Very helpful for anyone who experiences distracting thoughts, helping women to orgasm but also allowing men to slow down ejaculation too.

It releases anger from the heart and discharges feelings of unworthiness and not being enough. I find this especially useful for anyone intimidated by authority, new job, new boss etc which of course can easily translate into secondary sexual problems.

Celery Seed also reconditions attitudes about fatherhood and relationships with older men. Here we see themes rather than specifics, so we might think, new dad not coping, man worried about impregnating or not impregnating his partner, sexual abuse, emotional abuse, feelings of inadequacy...the list is endless.

Finally, I think it is worth going back to the word intimidated...which could be appropriate in any context, and celery seed would be helpful.

Physically for new mums, celery seed encourages milk flow.

Blending Note: Top

Blends Well With:

Top Note: Angelica, Bergamot, Melissa, May Chang & Lemon Verbena

Heart Note: Lavender, Rosemary, Basil,

Base Note: Jasmine and Myrrh

Cinnamon
Cinnamomum zeylanicum

Cinnamon is hot and fiery and, since it is a dermal irritant, is probably best avoided in most topical treatments. Diffused or burnt though, it brings sanctity to a space, clearing negative vibrations and creating a blank canvas. It releases anger and lets it just drift away.

Cinnamon speaks to cells of the body holding sad memories and asks them to melt away. It allows for honest retrospection and motivates the spirit to move forward. It dissipates repeated relationship patterns, breaking cycles of behaviour.

It is passionate, sexual, and entrancing.

Blending Note: Middle to top

Character:

Hot, Cosy, Spicy, Sweet, Smoky, Mouth Wateringly Delicious!!!

Blends Well With:

Top Notes: Bergamot, Frankincense, Lemon & Orange

Heart Notes: Lavender, Rosemary, Thyme & Ylang Ylang

Base Notes: Myrrh, Sandalwood & Benzoin

Maximum Topical Dilution: 0.07%

Cautions: May interact with blood clotting and diabetes medications. Not suitable for use during pregnancy.

Clary Sage
Salvia sclarea

I have written an entire book about clary sage, so I won't labour on about it for too long! However, it such a relaxing oil and it is gorgeously euphoric. It has a heady feeling of lying down on the lawn and watching clouds on a summer's day.

Antispasmodic, it relaxes both physical tensions and emotional ones. On the most profound level, we might think of vaginosis where pain emanates from muscle tensions causing discomfort during sex.

Mentally, it lifts away stresses and strains, but it helps you to see more clearly too. If a relationship is sinking under the dust of arguments and misgivings, clary sage clears those away. Be aware that seeing clearly, of course, is the very opposite to the rose-coloured glasses of romance. But if confusion reigns, then clary sage is a massive help here.

Remember the effects of an essential oil are cumulative, so if the partnership is under strain, consider using this in a diffuser outside of the bedroom too. Give the air a chance to clear. Allow some opportunities to build bridges.

This is a glorious oil for couples who would like to become pregnant. Having oestrogen-like properties, it regulates the menstrual cycle and improves hormone levels. Physically it is a uterine tonic, giving the womb a thorough work out to get it into tip top shape.

That said, this oil comes with a few precautions:

No alcohol. Historically, it was used to adulterate beer, the flowers being cheaper than hops. The result is getting drunk and sleepy very fast and a very thick head in the morning! Standard advice would be not to use whilst working with heavy machinery, so watch the size of any saucy bed time toys! ☐

1. A uterine tonic and a mimic of oestrogen, this is a superb oil to get into shape for pregnancy. The slightest hope you might be pregnant, please stop using until 37 weeks when it will really help your labour along nicely. I usually advise taking six months off trying, use contraception and boost all levels with essential oils and take that opportunity enjoy sex together again. Then when you are ready to start trying again, omit topical use of some of the stronger oils like this one.

2. Clary Sage acts very strangely in peri-menopausal women. Since hormonal levels change so radically, in some cases clary sage can make mood swings and menstrual problems more problematic. If you find

this happens, I would recommend changing your choice to Chasteberry oil (*Vitex Agnus castus*).

Blending Note: Middle

It has a dry, musky fragrance that reminds me of cold tea! A bittersweet floral note, it is used extensively in perfumery as a fixative, making your blends last longer.

Blends Well With:

Top Notes: Grapefruit, Bergamot, Black Pepper, Lemon Balm, Lime, Mandarin, Cypress, Petitgrain,

Heart Notes: Bay, Cardamom, Chamomile, Coriander, Frankincense, Geranium, Jasmine, Juniper, Lavender, Pine, Rose, Tea Tree

Base Notes: Sandalwood, Patchouli, Cedarwood,

Maximum Dilution: 3%

Safety: Not suitable during first 37 weeks of pregnancy.

Frankincense
Boswellia carterii

For the most part frankincense is not aphrodisiac and yet is quintessential to sensuality. It slows the breath as if in tantric union. Moving your centre of being from the ego and into the body, frankincense centres emotional connection.

 It comforts and steadies, calming the haste of premature ejaculation.

It restores elasticity to relationships where the distance between a couple seems unassailable.

Blending Note: Top to Middle

Character: Resinous, Herbaceous, Pine-y, Opening, Comforting, Lifting, Reassuring, Connecting & Slowing

Blends well with:

Top Notes: Evergreen Notes, Pines, Firs & Spruces

Heart Notes: Herbaceous Lavenders, Rosemary & Sage

Base Notes: Resins & Woods

Maximum Dilution 3%

Cautions: *Not suitable for topical use during first 16 weeks of pregnancy.*

Galbanum
Ferula galbaniflua

Glorious, pacifying galbanum is like a warm comforting blanket scaring aware the darkest of shadows. Probably the most powerful of oils for somatic distress, it unblocks memories and allows a person to see how their "condition" has involved into what it has become. More, it gently helps them to face it in a safe and courageous fashion. Where it uncovers sadness and wrong doing, it is very much an oil of grace. Releasing the emotion gently, it lets the memory go. Perfect for panic attacks and restlessness, it allows a person to submit to their sexuality and lose themselves safely in the relaxation.

My feelings about galbanum as an aphrodisiac are very aligned to those I have about Holy Basil. Ocimum sanctum (Holy Basil) is *sattvic*, meaning perfect peace, and nothing sattvic should be ever used for sex. That's ayurvedic law. Hence, it is perfect for solving stress issues, but not for using as an aphrodisiac; it is consecrated and solemn. Galbanum, conversely is an equally hallowed medicine being used in many sacred incenses for thousands of years, but this *is* an aphrodisiac. That sense of peace is perfectly aligned to sex, but, not just any sex. This is an oil of profound union, for the deep intimacy of the heiro gamos, the esoteric marriage. We'll have no galbanum quickies around here! Respect please, where it is due.

Blending Note: Base

Character: Masculine, Pure, Seductive, Smokey, Delightful & Profound

Blends well with:

Top Notes: Bergamot, Cypress, Frankincense, Pines

Heart Notes: Geranium, Lavender, Clary Sage

Base Notes: Cedarwood & Myrrh

Maximum Dilution: 3%

Cautions: *Not suitable for topical use during first 16 weeks of pregnancy. Old oils are subject to high levels of oxidation, so replace bottles regularly to avoid risk of skin sensitisation.*

Geranium (Rose)

Pelargonium graveolens

Beautiful flower to end all flowers, in my opinion. She is cheerful and gentle, playful, and relaxing. She lifts the day's stress off the shoulders as if it were never there. Hormonally balancing she eases PMT and the symptoms of menopause, and balances male reproduction.

Where other oils linger and expect praise, geranium just delivers and moves onto something else. A very pragmatic oil, she is the perfect oil for absolutely every team. She recognises opportunities and threats in situations and finds ways for you to navigate them. On one hand she feels like she has no spiritual dimension of the other she feels like she *is* the spiritual realm, a guardian angel, if you will. There is something about her that instils resourcefulness and sparks something unusual and vital inside.

Anything that rose can do, geranium can do with less fuss! She deals with issues of abandonment and heartache. Where rose will sit calmly by holding your hand while you cry, geranium says "Well this won't get things done will it? Let's multiskill..." and she lifts you from the worries and says here, get on with things while you think. She finds solutions, but in a way that create them from that sacred space within you.

So, geranium is aphrodisiac but not in a glamorous hearts and flowers way. She's the perfect oil for every day sex, for loving each other when times are kicking you in the teeth, for tired days and irritated evenings. But, for goodness sake don't mistake he as less than important, as such this makes her the absolutely *most* important. Geranium is the cement that holds sanity together.

Blending Note: Middle

Character: Floral, Sweet, Happy, Romantic, Balancing, Sustaining, Restorative & Relaxing.

Blends well with:

Top Notes: Spices & Citruses

Heart Notes: Florals & Herbs

Base Notes: Woods & Resins...oh and blissfully clings to vetiver!

Maximum Dilution 3%

Cautions: *Not suitable in the first 16 weeks of pregnancy.*

Ginger
Zingiber officinale

Warming and soothing ginger is the perfect way to cut through feelings of powerlessness. Here, we might think about worries of impotence, or the stress that comes from being trapped in situations outside of your control.

It cuts through sensations of being victimised and impowers you to stand up to challenges in life. Creating inner fire it instils the courage to step into the role of leader inside of the bedroom and outside, in the wider world.

Physically it is stimulating, chasing away lethargy and apathy, making you stand alert! Emotionally, though, it balances, teaching a sweet spot between courage and fear and worries about scarcity and abundance. Bringing you very much into the present, it helps to appreciate what you have now, not worry about what is to come.

Obviously, the oil is extracted from the root and with all medicines taken this way, it is grounding, invigorating to the self, enabling you to find / remember who you are.

In Ayurveda ginger, is *rajasic*, promoting change through irritation. It is like a bolt from the blue shocking the emotional body into the physical.

Physically, it settles digestive problems and UTIs, clearing tension and soreness.

Blending Note: Middle

Character: Warm, Spicy, Comforting, Stimulating, Invigorating & Cossetting

Blends well with:

Top Notes: Citruses, Frankincense & Black Pepper

Heart Notes: Cardamom, Ylang Ylang, Cinnamon, Caraway, Geranium, Eucalyptus, Peppermint.

Base Notes: Woods & Resins

Maximum Dilution 3%

Cautions: *Not suitable in the first 16 weeks of pregnancy.*

Hyacinth
Hyacinthus orientalis

An expensive and rare absolute, there are rumblings in the industry that no true hyacinth oil exists. I'm too spellbound to care. The narcotic fragrance of hyacinths fills our garden in April, heralding the end of the winter and the hope of the new year to come. It echoes the ancient Greek belief that hyacinth brings the end of emotional winter, and gathers-in the spring.

Her ancient name is "Sorrow Flower" probably from this Greek connotation, but also because she is one of the forefront essences to treat grief. A comforting friend to those who struggle to express themselves, because their load is too heavy to bear. She is reassuring and consoling, distancing a person from their loss.

Physically, she is especially good at unwinding stress in the neck and shoulder mantle, and as the oils penetrate the skin, they circulate to the brain where she activates right brain thinking: creativity, imagination and seeing. Narcotic, she is sweet and inviting, lulling the scented to sleep. A potent (although costly) antidote to insomnia, hyacinth wards off unpleasant dreams.

Aphrodisiac, in the very strongest fashion, hyacinth is an oil for the broken- hearted.

Blending Note: Top

Character: Soft, Green, Floral, Honeyed, Narcotic, Reassuring, Comforting & Sweet.

Blends Well With:

Top Notes: Lemon Fragranced Citruses

Heart Notes: Violet, Ylang Ylang, Jasmine, Neroli

Base Notes: Amyris, Ambrette, Cedarwood, Myrrh

Maximum Dilution: 1.3%

Cautions: *Not suitable in the first 16 weeks of pregnancy.*

Jasmine

Jasminum officinale

Where rose is the symbol of love in the West, Jasmine is its counterpart in the East. Throughout the Himalayas, she is regarded as love, sensuality, and spiritual awakening. At Indian weddings, garlands of jasmine are offered to the Kama in a request that the couple's love will endure.

Jasmine balances turbulent emotions, allowing a person to think out their problems in a peaceful, tranquil space. Somehow worries seem to drift away on the ether as jasmine increases alpha brainwaves, settling thoughts.

The oil lets people face their dilemmas bravely and is the powerful yang energy of directed action, even when the body and spirit are most tired. It balances the chakras, in particular, the pineal, opening clearer sight into one's problems but also at the sacral, rooting and grounding a person.

This is an exquisite oil to choose if the sensuality has waned because of a dislike of one's body image. If sexuality and allure seem like things of the past, jasmine coaxes it back, reassuring and building self-esteem.

Enlarges male sexual organs and reduces prostate glands.

Unusually, jasmine is aphrodisiac and supporting to both men and women and is the perfect oil to add to masculine blends. Nevertheless, her energy connects to the feminine, empowering women and softening emotions in men.

Dissipating nervous tension, it instils feelings of optimism and happiness for the future. It is the must have oil in an any seduction box.

Blending Note: Middle

Character: Sensuous, Sweet, Inviting, Reflective, Tranquil, Comforting & Balancing.

Blends Well With:

Top Notes: Lemon! The most sublime mix!

Heart Notes: Florals & Spices.

Base Notes: Resins

Maximum Dilution 3%

Cautions: *Not suitable for use during pregnancy until after 37 weeks.*

Labdanum
Cistus labdanum

In some ways labdanum and galbanum seem interchangeable here, but if I had to cite a difference, labdanum feels more acute to me. That feeling of cartoon cat, where the terror is so keen that it makes conscious decision making impossible. Where galbanum is for the afraid or anxious, labdanum is for the scared witless.

There is a sense of immediate dread here, but this is one of the quintessential choices for trauma (along with amber.) It uncovers old hurts and brings forward buried memories, bringing spiritual experiences into the conscious mind.

Labdanum (or rock rose) quietens the mind and brings about a rather energised calm. Where galbanum brings about blissful surrender, labdanum smiles, "right then, let's do this". It's mysterious and masculine and blends beautifully to balance female scents.

I think it is worth noting the plant thrives on neglect. Thus, this might be a good oil to start with if your relationship has not had any TLC for a while. Somehow it feels less arcane than galbanum, so you can probably use it a bit more freely for every day sex.

Blending Note: Base

Character: *Recollecting, dissipating, cajoling, reassuring, rescuing, sedative*

Blends Well With:

Top Notes: Angelica, Cypress, Pine, Frankincense

Heart Notes: Lavender, Clary Sage

Base Notes: Sandalwood, Patchouli, Vetiver

Maximum Dilution: 3%

Cautions: *Not suitable for topical use during first 16 weeks of pregnancy.*

Lavender
Lavandula angustifolia

In itself, lavender is not aphrodisiac, but there is a great deal to be said for being calm and relaxed. Add in small amounts to blends.

Blending Note: Heart or Middle

Character: Floral, Herbaceous, Aromatic.

Blends Well With:

Top Notes: Lemon, Bergamot, Lemongrass, Angelica, Mandarin

Heart Notes: Rosemary, Basil, Rose, Geranium

Base Notes: Vetiver, Myrrh, Sandalwood, Cedarwood.

Maximum Dilution: 3%

Cautions: Not suitable for topical use during first 16 weeks of pregnancy: Not suitable before 16 weeks of pregnancy.

Lemon
Citrus x limonum

I always thought one of the most exotic and romantic tales I ever heard was that of Scheherazade, who beguiled the sultan with stories over 101 nights to protect herself from being beheaded. The Sultan became enchanted with her stories and fascinated with the woman herself. It's a strange a eloquent love story and yet I think a dimension that is missing from 21st century love affairs. When we pledge a lifetime together, how do we keep our partner interested?

Strangely, it is hard to sense whether lemon should be called he or she, the vibration of the oil is slightly garrulous and camp. It is energetic and open, inspiring creativity and intellect. Lemon always reminds me of Scheherazade, no sense of frailty or vulnerability, incredibly brave, outspoken and forthright. Not a cloud in the sky, bright tailed and perky, always a smile every single day. And when tomorrow comes, a different story to tell.

Physically we know the oil exerts a profound effect on the body's mood modulator serotonin. It enlivens us, lifts, and cheers us. It is clever little oil with plenty to say.

On its own, Lemon is not aphrodisiac, but like most top notes that stimulate our mental faculties, she blends gorgeously with more obviously seductive oils like jasmine and rose to seduce and entice via the old grey matter.

Blending Note: Top

Character: Bright, Pervasive, Sweet, Sharp, Happy & Bracing.

Blends Well With:

Top Notes: Citruses, Neroli, Petitgrain

Heart Notes: Roman Chamomile, Elemi, Frankincense, Rose, Ylang Ylang

Base Notes: Sandalwood

Maximum Dilution: 3%

Cautions: *Not suitable for topical use during first 16 weeks of pregnancy.*

Mandarin
Citrus auriantum

It's useful that lemon and mandarin sit so closely together in this book since she exerts that same brain cell seduction as the yellow fruit but...

Mandarin is a specific for the adrenal glands. These, more than any other part of the body suffer the effects of stress and, over long periods of pressure, will eventually become exhausted. When this happens, they leech power from organs like the liver and particularly the pituitary glands impeding the production of sex hormones and making libido wane.

If there are issues with stress, libido, impotence, or any kind of sexual debility gorgeous mandarin is a must have in the blend.

Blending Note: Top

Character: Happy, Sensible, Sustaining, Discrete, Adaptable & Generous

Blends well with:

Top Notes: Citruses & Spices

Heart Notes: Rose, Geranium, Chamomile, in particular, as well as spices, including the important relationship with the pituitary support of Nutmeg.

Base Notes: Vetiver, Myrrh, Woods And Importantly Sesquiterpene Rich Cedarwood.

Maximum Dilution 3%

Cautions: *Not suitable in the first 16 weeks of pregnancy.*

Mimosa

Acacia dealbata

A gorgeously bonding oil that mends breaks in families and creates closer unions. It is aphrodisiac, but extends further making it an oil to be diffused to heal family rifts generally.

Mimosa is a playfully happy place, it's a space that shows what lies behind. It's the colours in the sunrise, the smile inside of the laughter, the layer below if you like. There is something protective about mimosa, like drifting on angel's wings when you sleep, relaxing into those enormously safe feathers when entirely frazzled by life.

Mimosa moves experience from the mental realm to the heart, she inspires forgiveness and compassion, stripping away what went before and turning back the clock.

Strangely, witches believe that mimosa life releases you from a hex, and I do feel it unlocks the shackles of curses you feel cast shadows over your bed.

It calms hypersensitivity, so that's an incredible boon to relationships teetering on the edge. Somehow, it lifts you away, releasing frayed feelings into the wind.

It attracts love, and being ruled as a water element, promotes the flow of emotion. It encourages forgiveness and increases lust.

Blending Note: Middle to Top

Character: Soothing, Uplifting, Smiling, Binding, Pervasive (aroma, so use sparingly!) & Sumptuous.

Blends well with:

Top Notes: Bergamot, Neroli

Heart Notes: Coriander, Rose, Petitgrain, Star Anise

Base Notes: Amyris, Cedarwood & Agarwood.

Cautions: *Not suitable for topical use during first 16 weeks of pregnancy*

Myrrh
Commiphora myrrha

Of all the plants in the Bible, none is mentioned more often than myrrh, and it is usually used there in the context of seduction.

> *My beloved is to me a sachet of myrrh resting between my breasts.*
>
> **Song of Solomon 1-13**

To me, if there is any kind of sexual dysfunction, then you probably do need to be using myrrh. Emotionally, it releases feelings of being stuck. Bringing up hidden feelings and hang ups, it removes the need for control, releases distrust and enhances intimacy.

It's an incredibly protecting oil to the skin and tissues and this extends into the emotional realm where it seems to make you want to wrap your arms around your lover and take care of them.

It purifies the aura enabling hurts and wounds to heal. Certainly, this oil is consecrated, but it seems allied to a sacredness of the human form and sexual union. Transforming negative energy, myrrh amplifies the power of any other oils in its blend.

It is cooling, and of course, is one of the base note fixatives in blends whose medicine will linger on you long after you have climbed out of bed.

Blending Note: Base

Character: Seductive, Healing, Creative, Destructive, & Enticing

Blends well with:

Top Notes: Lemongrass, Citronella, Lemon, Orange, Frankincense

Heart Notes: Tea Tree, Eucalyptus, Geranium, Cypress, Juniper, Palma Rosa

Base Notes: Patchouli

Maximum Dilution: 3%

Cautions: *Not suitable for topical use during first 37 weeks of pregnancy*

Neroli

Citrus aurantium subsp. amara

This oil comes from flowers of orange trees and was given its name after an Italian princess of Nerola. Anne Marie de la

Trémoille (Orsini), a duchess of Bracciano first introduced society to orange blossom when she created her own fashionable signature scent by bathing in it, perfuming her stationary, scarves and most famously, her gloves.

In China, it is the traditional flower carried at weddings symbolising purity, chastity, and innocence. Embracing symbology plays a big part in creating aphrodisiacs, and we can see that a neroli fragrance doesn't really marry up with black stockings and suspenders. This is a gentle night, tender, slow and loving.

In Victorian times, it was accepted that every bridal bouquet would include orange blossom, partly for very practical reasons since many weddings took place in the early summer, it was guaranteed flowers would be available. But this idea of may also have came from 19th century society mags who had seen Queen Victoria carry an enormous bouquet down the aisle to marry Prince Albert.

Orange blossom is revered in China, for its predictability to produce prolific numbers of fruits at the same time every year. Thus, orange blossom also symbolises fertility and a fruitful marriage. Several Victorian papers show prudish writers finding the link between the delicate flowers and fertility utterly obscene, which tickles the hell out of me, especially since their monarch seemed to be making a good example of the fact it could very well have been so! Incidentally, if you're looking for beautiful fragrances to blend with it, rosemary and myrtle were often woven through the blossoms in head dresses and the scent is exquisite.

Medicinally, anxiety is one of the primary oils we use for anxiety. It is calming, pacifying and reassuring.

Blending Note: Top to Middle

Light, sweet-floral fragrance redolent of oranges! Blend with care because delicate neroli can often disappear in heavy mixes.

Character: Romantic, Whimsical, Light, Coy, Charming & Alluring.

Blends well with:

Top Notes: Bergamot, Petitgrain,

Heart Notes: Geranium, Lavender & Rose,

Base Notes: Peru Balsam, Myrrh, Agarwood, Cedarwood, Sandalwood & Vanilla

Maximum dilution 3%

Cautions: Not suitable for topical use in the first 16 weeks of pregnancy

Nutmeg
Myristica fragrans

Another neglected oil, in my opinion, and the quintessential choice for impotence and loss of libido.

This top note fuels the sagging pituitary during stress, fortifying hormonal flow.

Emotionally, it forgives betrayal and loss, and comforts the solar plexus in trauma. Energising the flow of energy through the body it unwinds blockages at the abdomen and sex organs. Drawing energy upward from the root chakra to the core, it activates kundalini, increasing fire and spirit.

Nutmeg absolves doubt and resistance, allowing you to take a plunge into the unknown. Where other oils might release hurts, nutmeg seems to carry them for you, sympathetic and accepting, simply supporting until you are ready to let go. This is an oil that understands healing take time and yet life still has to go on.

Nutmeg, for many, is the first step towards happiness.

Blending Note: Strong Middle to Top

 (Be careful it doesn't overwhelm the scent of the rest of your blend.)

Character: Punchy, Aggressive, Forceful, Potent, Stabilising & Fiery.

Blends Well With:

Top Notes: Bergamot, Citruses & Evergreens

Heart Notes: Lavender, Rose, Mimosa, Petitgrain, Clary Sage, Cypress

Base Notes: Patchouli & Vetiver

Maximum Dilution

Cautions: *Not suitable for topical use during first 16 weeks of pregnancy*

Orange

Citrus sinensis

I think it was Valerie Ann Worwood who first said orange carries sunlight and the radiance of the stars. Beautifully eloquent. Orange has a very high healing energy and is profoundly connected to self-confidence. I'd say there were two specific types of people here that orange will help. Those who obsess over perfection, and those who struggle to relinquish control.

If your mind wanders to how you look or what you should be doing next, orange will be an amazing tonic. Imagine that sensation of lying back and succumbing to the magic of space as you gaze up into the stars; there, is oranges glow.

The orange tree, as a whole, is profoundly connected to seduction, with blossoms being used as wedding bouquets and engagements. Indeed, magickal texts tell me that infusions of orange leaves and flowers might even get you a marriage proposal, but make what you will of that. Unmistakably though, it is alluring and inspiring and a regular drop or two added to potions and lotions increases beauty and attractiveness, and helps you to know it too.

Orange encourages adaptability and builds a more flexible attitude and that is a rich source of nourishment for lovers who have forgotten how to be friends. This is an oil of give and take, of lightness of heart and playfulness. Not childish, but yet childlike, innocent and hopeful, whimsical, frivolous and happy.

Blending Note: Top

Character: Confident, Feisty, Alluring, Upbeat, Decisive & Ambitious

Blends well with:

Top Notes: Spices & Citruses

Heart Notes: Geranium, Petitgrain, Neroli, Rose, Clary Sage, Frankincense, Rosemary, Basil

Base Notes: Patchouli, Sandalwood & Myrrh

Maximum Dilution

Cautions: *Not suitable for topical use during first 16 weeks of pregnancy.*

Patchouli
Pogostemon cablin

Patchouli is an extremely important sexual oil and might probably *the* most important one you can use to move forward from sexual difficulties. It is profoundly seductive, encouraging lusty urges, but this is almost the levels of tantric union, instilling sensations of the sacredness of life.

It stimulates the fount of femininity, opening receptiveness and awakening fertility. Building sexual potency, it tantalises the sensory levels and strokes the auric fields. Perception of time is slowed, so intercourse can just go on and on, and as it does there is a primordial sensation of merging as the spiritual body sinks into the physical self.

This is extraordinary healing for those detached from themselves; those who neglect their physical wellness and cannot perceive how that internal relationship is affecting how sensual they do or don't feel. Likewise, if the body relaxes, but the mind chatters on, patchouli gently turns the lights out quieting internal discourse and stilling internal thoughts. Patchouli brings about the most delicious unification of the self.

But for all its esoteric magic, patchouli is very sensible. Reasonable and practical it is very grounded medicine. Invigorating and stimulating it keeps the feet very firmly planted in reality; it helps to build far sightedness into an equation.

Just because we don't work now doesn't mean we can't be fixed.

When I use patchouli, I always get a sense of the times of Raj, and of the women that went over with their husbands to serve. While they take tea, they are civilised, pragmatic, cool and alluring and that's exactly how patchouli works. Its relaxed but not flighty. Voluptuous but modest. Strong and yet vulnerable too.

Blending Note: Middle to Base (Very potent aroma)

Character: Sensual, Paradoxical, Refined, Sensible, Imaginative & Gracious.

Blends well with:

Top Notes: Bergamot, Lemon, Orange, Melissa

Heart Notes: Lavender, Rose, Geranium, Clary Sage, Jasmine, Palmarosa, Petitgrain

Base Notes: Myrrh, Sandalwood, Amyris

Maximum Dilution: 3%

Cautions: Not suitable for topical use during first 16 weeks of pregnancy:

Rose

Rosa damascena

The most romantic of all the oils, rose is crowned queen. I find *damascena* a little more prosaic than *centrifolia*, as if wife were being compared to courtesan. Both are alluring, enigmatic, seductive, and healing but one a little more mysterious, adept, and aloof.

I find it very hard to write about rose because I am aware she is a book in herself. I know that, I wrote it! And the most exquisite part of the research I did, was into her effects on male sexuality, how she rebuilds and repairs not only the emotional fall out of depression but also the after effects of the drugs men have to take to feel happier too. After a few weeks of using rose not only did their libido return but their erections, orgasms, and ejaculations did too. Truly, if you are struggling with sexual problems, you should definitely read that book.

But rose is connected to the heart chakra, and while I probably have overlooked that aspect of sexuality for the most part in this book, it cannot be ignored here. If the heart aches from pain, that will find its way to the bedroom. Rose is the perfect medicine.

Physically too, it is a uterine tonic, affecting fertility and hopefully aiding pregnancy.

Blending Note: Middle to Top

Character: Romantic, Steadying, Uplifting, Soothing, Feminine, & Nostalgic.

Blends well with:

Top Notes: Spices & Citruses

Heart Notes: Clary Sage, Neroli, Lavender, Camomile, Coriander

Base Notes: Myrrh, Vetiver & Sandalwood

Maximum Dilution 3%

Cautions: *Not suitable for topical use during first 37 weeks of pregnancy:*

Sandalwood
Santalum album

Where rose is queen, then sandalwood is her most faithful courtier; together they work through the heart chakra stimulating sexual activity and combatting fear. Sandalwood seems to act like the guardian of the bed chamber, consecrating it as sacred space. Encouraging emotional openness in partnerships, it breaks old habits and thought patterns, rejuvenating the unity two people once felt together.

Sandalwood promotes honesty in discourse and supports togetherness and stability. Its woody energy allows dappled light of hope to shine through the trees, opening it up to radiant sunshine when all else feels like winter around.

Breathe sandalwood to release negativity and to guide distractions to the back of your mind. Encouraging receptivity, this fleshy base note reopens the sensual joys of the body.

Blending Note: Base

Character: Sensuous, Profound, Meditative, Consecrating & Rejuvenating

Blends well with:

Top Notes: Bergamot, Lemon Verbena, Grapefruit.

Heart Notes: Cypress, Frankincense, Juniper, Jasmine. Rose, Lavender, Ylang Ylang

Base Notes: Cedarwood, Labdanum & Vetiver

Maximum Dilution 3%

Cautions: *Not suitable for topical use during first 16 weeks of pregnancy*

Spikenard
Nardostachys jatamansi

This is the oil of the most scared and afraid, and again, is a book I have previously written. Again, to me this feels like an oil too precious to use. It's not an oil for sex; it is a medicine for life saving surgery. If something that has shattered you or a loved one to core, then spikenard is the electric shock that brings you back from hell. I guess we are talking about affairs, death of children, rape, PTSD... read this with your life story. You fill in the blanks.

It settles aftershocks and helps you face down your most terrifying thoughts. Releasing fear of the unknown, jatamansi reconciles you, making peace. It balances emotions and instils a sense of devotion bringing about the most revered forgiveness.

Spikenard is divine intervention when clemency might never otherwise be explained.

Blending Note: Base

Character: Forgiving, Steadying, Fortifying, Accepting & Acquiescent

Blends Well With:

Top Notes: Clove, Frankincense, Ginger & Angelica Seed

Heart Notes: Juniper, Rose, Geranium & Lavender

Base Notes: Myrrh & Vetiver

Maximum Dilution: 3%

Cautions: Not suitable for topical use during first 16 weeks of pregnancy.

Star Anise
Illicium verum

Here we take a little break from the deeply arcane oils into simple spice. Anise brings about a more harmonious space but also reminds partners how to love consciously. Its warming embrace melts those most resistant to change, and calms anxiety about the future.

Traditional Chinese Medicine suggests drinking a glass of warm water infused with the seeds each day to increase libido. I must confess to have become rather an addict of them in warm milk in the evening and it does seem to add a certain *je ne sais quoi* to my day! They are not astoundingly mind-blowing medicine, but they do instil warmth and contentedness and in some ways, that is all of us could ever wish for. It is soft, comforting, and entwining medicine.

Blending Note: Middle

Character: Spicy, Exotic, Snuggly, Harmonious, Flexible & Accommodating.

Blends well with:

Top Notes: Orange, Neroli, Cypress, Lime & Nutmeg

Heart Notes: Camomile, Rose, Fennel & Peppermint

Base Notes: Myrrh, Vanilla & Amyris

Maximum Dilution 1.7%

Cautions: *Not suitable for topical use during pregnancy or whilst breastfeeding.*

Tuberose
Polianthes tuberosa

Tuberose was sacred to the Maya, as a means of communicating with their divine entities, believing it to connect them with sacred creativity. The glorious white Polianthes flower is pure dangerous pleasure. Voluptuous, enticing and tempting, the Hindus refer to this wanton harlot as the Queen of The Night. The French warn against young girl being allowed to smell her scent after dark lest they become consumed by feelings of ardour and lust.

There is a sybaritic oozing of sexiness with tuberos,e as you feel the energies engorging your chakras and vital organs. You feel more appealing, bursting, and full of ardour. And yet she acts like a curtain. She conceals secrets you would never want anyone to know, like impotence, frigidity, or pain, holding you in her ecstatic embrace. She is urgent, passionate, and lusty.

She understands things might not be great, that perhaps you feel insecure, jealous of resentful and yet says "F**k it, let's just do it anyway". Then, letting you pass behind the curtain she hides your own worries and inadequacies from even you, allowing you to get on with the job in hand.

Physically, she is antispasmodic to both muscles and nerves and engorges extremities with blood flow. Normally, I might suggest it doesn't really matter where on the body you use the oil, but I think the more focused you can be with tuberose, the more intensely you will feel her pleasure.

Of all the oils designed to be aphrodisiac, tuberose is probably the one blending gorgeously with all the other usual suspects of rose, sandalwood, jasmine, and patchouli.

Blending Note: Middle to top

Character: Slutty, lascivious, voluptuous, enticing and seducing

Top Notes: Bergamot, Neroli, Orange & Petitgrain

Heart Notes: Clary Sage, Lavender, Rose, Mandarin

Base Notes: Patchouli, Sandalwood & Vetiver

Maximum Dilution 1.2%

Cautions: *Not suitable for topical use during first 16 weeks of pregnancy.*

Vetiver

Vetiveria zizanoides

Sex...relax...action...get on with it. Enough said!

Vetiver has no interest in the whys and wherefores. He's a quiet, stable creature that demands you just get on with it. He makes it easier to concentrate and hold your attention in your body, he slows sensation down and fortifies internal energy. Blissful, easy, and sensuous.

Blending Note: Base

Character: Masculine, Sensual, Focused, Directing, Purifying & Sanctifying.

Blends well with:

Top Notes: Citruses, Neroli, Petitgrain

Heart Notes: Rose, Clary Sage, Jasmine, Lavender, Mandarin, Ylang Ylang

Base Notes: Patchouli, Sandalwood & Cedarwood.

Maximum Dilution

Cautions: *Not suitable for topical use during first 16 weeks of pregnancy.*

Ylang ylang
Cananga odorata

The Madagascan Flower of Flowers is spread over bridal beds on wedding nights. A wonderful oil for addressing sexual anxiety, its relaxing and euphoric medicine lulls the user into exotic bliss.

Ylang ylang has a theme of balancing. Balancing hormones, balancing skin combinations, blood pressure etc. Here it also balances emotions and to some extent it is very clever at treating people to a taste of their own medicine. Its fragrance can be cloying and suffocating and seems to balance suffocating emotions like jealousy, possessiveness, the dark sides of wanting to care for someone.

It integrates the feminine divine, and perhaps that may be how the seesaw tips, as self-esteem is lifted by her scent, the desire to hold quite so tightly seems to let go.

Ylang ylang says: "Take a step back. Relax. Lie back. And just trust, because I assure you, everything is just going to be OK."

Blending Note: Middle

Character: Super-Sweet (Bordering on Nauseating), Harmonising, Balancing, Uplifting, Sedating, Languid and Luxuriating.

Blends well with:

Top Notes: Citruses, Nutmeg & Black Pepper

Heart Notes: Frankincense, Clary Sage, Geranium, Rose, Jasmine

Base Notes: Myrrh & Vetiver

Maximum Dilution: 1%

Cautions: *Not suitable for topical use during first 37 weeks of pregnancy*

Yuzu
Citrus junos

Many of the oils we use to still the mind are base notes, drawing energy *down*wards. Yuzu is the exception that proves the rule. She drives energy up, focusing it, divesting penetrating precision and awareness.

She allows us to look past our annoyances and worries. She is uplifting, optimistic and joyous and yet peaceful.

Strictly (or loosely) speaking she is not an aphrodisiac oil, but one cannot overlook its extraordinary anti-depressant effects which doubtless have a bearing on sexuality.

Blending Note: Top

Character: Uplifting, Directing, Focusing, Positive, Bright & Calm.

Blends well with:

 Top Notes: Basil & Petitgrain

(Not citruses, the fragrance disappears.)

Heart Notes: Roman Camomile, Clary Sage, Frankincense, Geranium, Ylang Ylang & Rose

Base Notes: Patchouli, Sandalwood & Vetiver

Maximum Dilution 3%

Cautions: *Not suitable for topical use during first 16 weeks of pregnancy.*

Zdravets
Geranium macrorrhizum L.

I am rather smug to see this oil becoming more popular because Cranesbill geraniums grow like weeds in my garden. The Strong Silent One curses them, popping up everywhere, but I adore them they are so romantically pretty. Long used in Traditional Bulgarian Medicine, they are aphrodisiac and anti-spasmodic.

Even though it is unrelated to our aromatherapy geranium, *Pelargonium graveolens,* Zdravets does tend to mimic her effects then ramp them up on steroids; über relaxing, incredibly merry and a very good hormonal balancer to boot.

Blending Note: Middle

Blends Well With:

Top Note: Citruses and Spices

Heart Note: Geranium, Rose, Lavender, Monarda

Base Note: Vetiver.

Chapter 5 Essential Oil Recipes for Aphrodisiac Blends
Reader, if this is the first one of my books you have read, please also download your free copy of The Complete Guide to Clinical Aromatherapy and The Essential Oils of The Physical Body, from Amazon to learn how to use essential oils and basic blending. This is not covered here, in this book.

In some ways this chapter of recipes completely undo the whole idea of the book, that you create your own blends based on yours and your partner's needs, but since so many of you love them...

Here are your starting points and then you can tweak and adjust them. (Somehow that sounds a tad risqué in the context of this book...!)

I do think there is such a thing as sensory overload with essential oils, so I suggest choosing a couple of blends and using the oils in them as themes throughout the house. Imagine the effect of someone wearing five or six bottles of perfume at one time...it is just too much and too many different fragrances in the home can certainly do the same. Subtlety is the name of the game here,

I've created formulae, based on the obvious themes of the issues, but when you read the oils back again, I'm sure you'll go "that's what I need" then you can swap and change oils in and out as you go.

Try to keep the synergy going here. If you take out a Top Note, see if you can replace with the same. If you can maintain the inverted pyramid of ratios (3 drops Top Note, 2 drops Heart Notes, 1 drop Base Note) I think you will find the magnificence of the blend swells here, since we really do want to harmonise body mind and spirit, rather than sticking a plaster on a purely physical wound.

Once you have created your master formula, you can transpose it into whatever aromatic format you like, whether that be a tablespoon of massage oil, 4oz bath salts or into candles.

The formulae are designed for diffusers and evaporators, but as I said, feel free to add to any base at all. I've added some ideas after the formulae.

The first five blends are for fun, no particular issues to deal with, just for more indulgent and wanton sex. Read further for help with upsetting conditions. Also, if you still struggle beyond the blends, you can find details of how to hire me as a consultant to create a blend especially for you and your partner, in the last section of this book.

A WARNING
Please be aware that no essential oil and condom relationship has ever ended well. Oils wreck latex and will compromise your birth control.

Peaceful Night In
- 3 drops Orange (*Citrus sinensis*)
- 2 drops Jasmine (*Jasminum officinale*)
- 1 drop Vetiver (*Vetiver zizanoides*)

Cautions: Not suitable for topical use during first 16 weeks of pregnancy: Not suitable for use in bath or massage during first 37 weeks of pregnancy.

Peaceful Night in For Pregnant Parents.
Suitable for all, but finding aphrodisiac oils that are safe to use topically during pregnancy is a challenge. This blend is only suitable after 16 weeks, but of course can be used in a diffuser all the way through and is also nice because it is full of anti-morning sickness oils! Before 16 weeks that I would suggest using thick luscious carriers for massage, omit the essential oils, and just leave the diffuser running.

- 3 drops Mandarin (*Citrus reticulata*)
- 2 drops Zdravets (Geranium macrorrhizum L)
- 1 drop Patchouli (*Pogostemon cablin*)

I remember you!
To reconnect after two many busy days.

- 1 drop Mandarin (*Citrus reticulata*)
- 1 drop Ylang Ylang (*Cananga Odorata*)
- 1 drop Cedarwood (*Cedrus atlantica*)

Cautions: Not suitable for topical use during first 16 weeks of pregnancy: Not suitable for use in bath or massage during first 37 weeks of pregnancy.

Ramp It Up a Notch
- 3 drops Yuzu (*Citrus junos*)
- 1 drop Ginger (*Zingiber officinalis*)
- 1 drop Clary Sage (*Salvia sclarea*)
- 1 drop Cinnamon (*Cinnamomum zeylanicum*)
- 1 drop Agarwood (*Aquilaria malaccensis*)

Slow It Down

- 3 drops Bergamot (*Citrus bergamia*)
- 2 drops Mimosa (*Acacia dealbata*)
- 1 drop Patchouli (*Pogostemon cablin*)

Intensity

- 3 drops Blue Lotus (*Nymphaea Caerulea*)
- 2 drops Jasmine (*Jasminum officinale*)
- 1 drop Sandalwood (*Santalum album*)

Open Communication

- 3 drops Yuzu (*Citrus junos*)
- 2 drops Ylang Ylang (*Cananga odorata*)
- 1 drops Amyris (*Amyris balsamifera*)

Impotence

- 3 drops Mandarin (*Citrus reticulata*)
- 2 drops Nutmeg (*Myristica fragrans*)
- 1 drop Jasmine (*Jasminum officinale*)

Low Sex Drive (Man)

- 3 drops Mandarin (*Citrus reticulata*)
- 2 drops Cardamom (*Elletaria cardomomum*)

- 1 drop Ginger (*Zingiber officinale*)
- 2 drops Jasmine (*Jasminum officinale*)

Low Sex Drive (Woman)
- 1 x Tuberose (*Polianthes tuberosa*)
- 1 x Rose (*Rosa centrifolia*)
- 1 x Sandalwood (*Santalum album*)

Too Busy Baby-Making to Be Lovers
- 3 x Orange (*Citrus sinensis*)
- 2 x Star Anise (*Illicium verum*)
- 1 x Patchouli (*Pogostemon cablin*)

Frigidity
- 1 x Tuberose (*Polianthes tuberosa*)
- 2 x Orange (*Citrus sinensis*)
- 2 x Clary Sage (*Salvia sclarea*)
- 3 x Jasmin (*Jasminum officinale*)

Premature Ejaculation
- 1 drop Orange (*Citrus sinensis*)
- 2 drops Rose geranium (*Pelargonium graveolens*)
- 3 drops Cedarwood atlas (*Cedrus atlantica*)
- 1 drop Patchouli (*Pogostemon cablin*)
- 1 drop Vetiver (*Vetiveria zizanoides*)

Delayed Orgasm
- 3 drops Yuzu (*Citrus junos*)

- 2 drops Blue lotus (*Nymphaea Caerulea*)
- 1 drop Rose (*Rosa damascena*)
- 2 drop Tuberose (*Polianthes tuberosa*)
- 2 drops Jasmin (*Jasminum officinale*)

Let's Connect on A Deeper Level
- 3 x Lemon (*Citrus limonum*)
- 2 x Frankincense (*Boswellia carterii*)
- 1 x Patchouli (*Pogostemon cablin*)

Setting the Scene.

People, I am a Cancerian. If there is something I know about it is nostalgic romance. Here's what my perfect evening looks like. Take influences from mine but make the night your own. Think about what would make the evening quintessentially yours and meld it to create a spell-bounding dream.

Wash and launder dinner table linen prior to use, adding 10 drops of your formulae to the final rinse in the washer. Use a tablespoon of Epsom salts in the middle compartment of the soap dispenser and drip the oils in. (Why not wash the bed linen at the same time for a matching fragrance and to save on oils, electric and water!)

Add 5 more drops of your blend into a teaspoon of vodka then into a spray bottle water to create a gorgeous ironing water too.

Using copious numbers candles (dinner and tealights) lay the table with beautiful glass-wear and silver to reflect the candlelight. Frost the rims of glasses by dipping them into lemon juice and then into sugar. Don't forget the most important a-romantic element, of course glorious perfumed flowers.

Perhaps nine and a half weeks is more your style, but for me a dinner of Morrocan Tagine with it gorgeous Eastern fragrances with a sticky cinnamon dessert. Then perhaps a rich cardamom latté to stimulate, although not too much. The cheekiest drip of rose or blue lotus into champagne guarantees a heady embrace.

Flirtatious Flickering Candles

I adore the delicate fragrance essential oils give to candles, far subtler than other ones you find in the shops. These look entirely exquisite on the dinner table and they are easy to make a batch at a time and store away until you need them.

The combinations and permutations are endless. You make the rules. So...

Buy a sheet of beeswax from the craft shop, from Ebay or direct from a beekeeper. They come in rectangles which will make four candles each.

- Cut the rectangle in half vertically and then cut each section diagonally to create two triangles.
- Smear your essential oils down the vertical edge of your triangle. I find about 3 drops of each works best per candle.
- Let it dry for a few moments then take a piece of cotton string to make a wick. Lay it along the same vertical side then crease a small line of the beeswax against the wick to hook it into place.
- Roll the beeswax snugly around the wick. Wind it as tightly as you can against the string. Trim the wick to length.

Don't put essential oil directly onto the wick because as they burn you lose the freshness of the scent.

Beguiling Tea Lights.
If you are not as nimble fingers, or if you are short on time then using plain old tea lights (plain white wax in a round foil container) work just as well. These are a really romantic way to add ambiance to the bedroom or bathroom (or how about a suggestive pathway up the stairs?

All you need to do is simply add essential oil to their melted wax. These are subtle and enticing, will cost you a fraction of the cost of store bough aromatherapy candles and since you have designed them entirely for your own relationship journey, they will be far more effective too.

The only difficult thing is controlling the wicks so....

Have some cocktail sticks at the ready!!

You say skillet, I say frying pan...Find the heaviest one you have, and ideally it will be the oldest and most battered you have!

With the stove burner turned *off*....

Fill your pan with as many candles as you can get in.

Pull all of your wicks up and very carefully lay cocktail sticks across the candle, either side of the wick to support it. You can even push it over to one side to prevent it from falling between them, if you are nervous.

When you are happy everything is secure, turn on the heat, very low.

The wax slowly turns to liquid, but it is easier to control the wicks if you don't let it completely melt all the way through.

When you are happy the wax is warm enough, turn off the heat and add about 5 drops of your blend to each candle.

Leave the pan where it is for the candles to set. This will ensure **you get a nice clean sheen to them.**

Irresistible Warm Flannels

There is something so sensuous about the warm flannels they give you in an Indian restaurant after dinner, although they are an enigma to me. How can they be so volcanically hot and then stone cold within seconds!!! They seem to defy physics!

Soak the flannel, squeeze out and fold.

Microwave on high for 30 seconds, then add 4 drops lemon essential oils.

Inviting Bathroom Towels

Add a tablespoon of Epsom Salts with your chosen formula, to the middle slot of your soap drawer in the washer. This will add oils to the final rinse of the wash.

I like to add the oils onto pieces of kitchen paper and fold them into the towels to keep fragrances subtle yet bright.

Mood Enhancing Massage oil

Blend the oils into 1 tsp sesame seed oil (*Sesame indicum)* and 1 tsp apricot kernel oil *(Prunus Armeniaca)*

Bewitching Bath salts

Add to 4oz Himalayan Sea Salts.

Seductive Silky Words

Add your formulae to a teaspoon of vodka and then add to a jar of ink. The alcohol dissolves the oils and fragrances your seductive notes and silvery tongued prose.

Conclusion

Essential oils are so much more than just a recipe and I hope you will have lots of fun experimenting and finding each other's fragrant trigger points together.

Hopefully, this will give you an opportunity to learn a whole new sensuality as a couple. Create new memories with your oils. Sensuality is so much more than just sex, it's about exploration, vulnerability ,and reflex. Get to know each other's loves and hates and explore vulnerable secrets that possibly no other partner will ever come to know.

It's a powerful tool and perhaps just one of the skills of the courtesan. Who knows, when you have mastered this, you'll take u wood work or buy a pole to dance round next!

I want to say a great big thank you to Kris Boggs who gave me the kick to do this book. It's one which has been flirting in my mind for months.

For the 3rd Birthday celebrations of The Secret Healer books, I invited questions for me to answer and Kris explained that she has many oils but doesn't feel she is very good at blending, so could I please design her a blend for her and her man and a quiet night in.

My mind chuntered round and around and I realised no cookie cutter blend would be good enough for the guys and gals who read my books. I owe you all so much for all your support and I wanted to gift you something truly unique.

 A voyage into aphrodisiacs; an uncommon way to explore yourself. The route to a happier, healthier, and more satisfied future. With love, from me, to you. - Liz

Get Better Acquainted with Elizabeth Ashley

Meet the Author

Elizabeth Ashley is an international speaker for the International Federation of Aromatherapists and the UK Director for the National Association of Holistic Aromatherapists. She is a prolific writer of professional articles, in particular for the IFA magazine Aromatherapy Thymes, Aromatika.hu, NAHA Journal and Holistic Therapist. She qualified as an aromatherapist in 1993, and then passed her Advanced Aromatherapy Diploma in 1994. She has been practicing aromatherapy for almost 25 years.

In 1999, she fell into a whole new career in the aggressive commercial sector of recruitment consultancy. There she discovered her father's second-hand car salesman genes had passed along and found she had quite the gift of the gab! More than that, she discovered she could sell...and then some.

In 2008, Elizabeth fell ill during pregnancy, with a blood clot in her lungs. The pulmonary embolism prevented her from working and she started to write. Very quickly, she gained her first contract as a ghost writer...a recipe book for cheese cakes!

In 2010, she was published professionally for her work on Galbanum - (*Ferula Galbaniflua*) oil in the Aromatherapy Thymes, journal of the International Federation of Aromatherapists, and on Tuberose (*Polianthes tuberosa*) oil by the New Zealand Register of Holistic Therapist.

In 2011, she was seconded on a consultative basis to Walsall Independent Treatment Centre, designed to be a rainbow bridge between traditional and complementary medicines. There she became aware of the rumblings of change in healthcare. Her book *Sales Strategies for Gentle Souls* explains the connotations of this.

Many of her books are aimed at helping qualified aromatherapists to expand their healing repertoire and build their businesses. She also writes for people who have an interest in essential oils and want to learn how to heal. Her in-depth essential oil profiles chart the healing properties of plants from the most arcane depths of historic folklore up to the scientific lab trials of today.

She lives in Shropshire with her husband and youngest son, kept company by their Staffordshire Bull Terrier, Bella, and many shoals of tropical fish! Her elder son and daughter have graduated from university this year (2017) and make her prouder than anything ever could. Elizabeth Ashley is The Secret Healer.

Consult with Me on Blending and Conditions
I offer a full consultancy service from one to one coaching over skype, with full case history, vitamin and essential oil therapies. Bespoke treatment formulae are created and sent to you as they need them. Journals and care plans provided. It's your personal therapist on demand.

Check out my new gig on **Fiverr** that will help you buy with confidence.

https://www.fiverr.com/elizabethstarns/l-will-check-your-essential-oil-blending

Perhaps you don't need the premium package. Maybe you know what oils you want to use but want reassurance you've picked safe ones. Again, I can help. Click the same link.

Hire me to write for you.

The marketplace is full of aromatherapy e-books written by people who have never so much as opened a bottle of essential oil. I know that because I learned to make cheesecakes from a book that I wrote! By contrast my books and articles are the culmination of twenty-five years professional experience and a lifetime of using aromatherapy,

If you want engaging content and well researched aromatherapy data, then contact me through my contractor page at Upwork.

https://www.upwork.com/o/profiles/users/_~01dabcae14e1938514/

Finally...

Are you a newcomer to aromatherapy and feel a bit bewildered or excited to learn more? Please feel free to get acquainted with a few basic oils.

Online Training from Me
93 videos about the fundamentals of aromatherapy and in-depth information on 15 different oils.

Find the course at:

https://beta.ofcourse.co.uk/course/aromatherapy-essential-oils-advanced

Normally priced at £199, please use discount code **TEACHER_ELIZA82** to get it for £35 (around $50) as a little thank you for all your support

Other Books by The Secret Healer

Book 1:- <u>The Complete Guide to Clinical Aromatherapy & Essential Oils for the Physical Body</u> (Free to download)

Book 2:- <u>Essential Oils for Mind Body Spirit</u>

Book 3:- <u>The Essential Oil Liver Cleanse</u>

Book 4:- <u>The Professional Stress Solution</u>

Book 5:- <u>The Aromatherapy Eczema Treatment</u>

Book 6:- <u>The Aromatherapy Bronchitis Treatment</u>

Book 7:- <u>50 Easy Recipes for Dry Skin</u>

Book 8:- <u>75 Easy Christmas Aromatherapy Recipes</u>

The Secret Healer Oils Profiles

1: <u>Monarda – A Native American Medicine</u>

2: <u>Vetiver – An Ayurvedic Medicine</u>

3: <u>Holy Basil – An Ayurvedic Medicine</u>

4: <u>Rose – Goddess Medicine</u>

5: <u>Sweet Basil – The Oil of Empowerment</u>

6: <u>Clary Sage- Natural Estrogen?</u>

7: <u>Spikenard- A Woman Washes Jesus's Feet. Was It our Oil of Aromatherapy?</u>

8: <u>Helichrysum – For The Wound That Will Not Heal</u>

9. Cannabis: How to Use the Cannabis Medicines of Aromatherapy.

Business Training for Professional Aromatherapists

Sales Strategies for Gentle Souls

Disclaimer

(1)   Introduction

This disclaimer governs the use of this eBook. By using this eBook, you accept this disclaimer in full. We will ask you to agree to this disclaimer before you can access the eBook.

(2)   Credit

This disclaimer was created using an <u>SEQ Legal</u> template.

(3)   No advice

The eBook contains information about aromatherapy and the use of essential oils. The information is not advice, and should not be treated as such.

You must not rely on the information in the eBook as an alternative to qualified medical advice from a health professional. If you have any specific questions about any medical matter you should consult an appropriately qualified professional.

If you think you may be suffering from any medical condition you should seek immediate medical attention. You should never delay seeking medical advice, disregard medical advice, or discontinue medical treatment because of information in this eBook.

(4)   No representations or warranties

To the maximum extent permitted by applicable law and subject to section 6 below, we exclude all representations, warranties, undertakings, and guarantees relating to the eBook. Without prejudice to the generality of the foregoing paragraph, we do not represent, warrant, undertake or guarantee:

> that the information in the eBook is correct, accurate, complete, or non-misleading;
> that the use of the guidance in the eBook will lead to any particular outcome or result; or
> in particular, that by using the guidance in the eBook you will heal disease or work in any way as a cure for illness.

(5)   Limitations and exclusions of liability

The limitations and exclusions of liability set out in this section and elsewhere in this disclaimer: are subject to section 6 below; and govern all liabilities arising under the disclaimer or in relation to the eBook, including liabilities arising in contract, in tort (including negligence), and for breach of statutory duty.

We will not be liable to you in respect of any losses arising out of any event or events beyond our reasonable control.

We will not be liable to you in respect of any business losses, including without limitation loss of or damage to profits, income, revenue, use, production, anticipated savings, business, contracts, commercial opportunities, or goodwill.

We will not be liable to you in respect of any loss or corruption of any data, database or software.

We will not be liable to you in respect of any special, indirect or consequential loss or damage.

(6) Exceptions

Nothing in this disclaimer shall: limit or exclude our liability for death or personal injury resulting from negligence; limit or exclude our liability for fraud or fraudulent misrepresentation; limit any of our liabilities in any way that is not permitted under applicable law; or exclude any of our liabilities that may not be excluded under applicable law.

(7) Severability

If a section of this disclaimer is determined by any court or other competent authority to be unlawful and/or unenforceable, the other sections of this disclaimer continue in effect.

If any unlawful and/or unenforceable section would be lawful or enforceable if part of it were deleted, that part will be deemed to be deleted, and the rest of the section will continue in effect.

(8) Law and jurisdiction

This disclaimer will be governed by and construed in accordance with English law, and any disputes relating to this disclaimer will be subject to the exclusive jurisdiction of the courts of England and Wales.

(9) Our details

In this disclaimer, "we" means (and "us" and "our" refer to) [*The Secret Healer)*] of [*4, SY8 1LQ)*].